S0-CKQ-784

The Complete Herbal Book
for the Dog

by the same author

*

HERBAL HANDBOOK FOR FARM AND STABLE
SUMMER IN GALILEE
HERBAL HANDBOOK FOR EVERYONE
NATURAL REARING OF CHILDREN

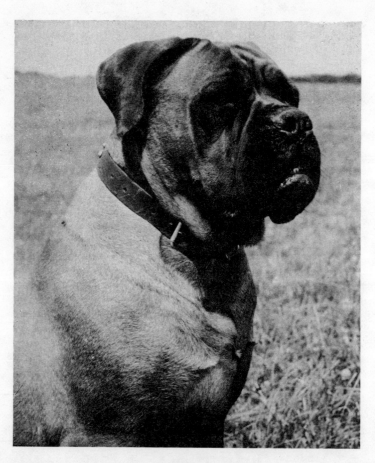

WYASTON ELIZABETH TUDOR

Bullmastiff. D. Oliff, Wyaston Kennels, Lydney, Gloucestershire. A superb bitch who has left her mark on the breed in many parts of the world, especially America and Canada. Bred of direct Wyaston lines by the author's friend, Douglas Oliff, who writes: 'In a breed where there is a high percentage of infertility amongst both bitches and dogs, my stock has never failed to produce offspring, which I attribute to their very natural surroundings (Forest of Dean), the raw foods diet, and no inoculations which has been a feature of the Wyastons for over seven generations of the same line. I am delighted to be in your book. As you know I have successfully followed your principles for so long now and put many other breeders on to them.' (*Photo: Douglas Oliff*)

THE COMPLETE HERBAL
BOOK FOR THE DOG

A Complete Handbook of Natural Care and Rearing

Juliette de Baïracli Levy

ARCO PUBLISHING COMPANY, INC.

New York

Third Printing, 1978

Published by Arco Publishing Company, Inc.
219 Park Avenue South, New York, N.Y. 10003

Copyright © 1971 by Juliette de Bairacli Levy

All rights reserved.

Library of Congress Catalog Card Number 72-3339
ISBN 0-668-02649-9 (Cloth Edition)
ISBN 0-668-04181-1 (Paper Edition)

Printed in United States of America

TO

MY TURKUMAN AFGHAN HOUNDS

who have wonderfully justified my belief in herbal
medicine and Nature method of canine rearing. Who
have never known disease and whose names, such as
Turkuman Bamboo, Turkuman Pomegranate, Turkuman Dammar Pine-tree, Turkuman Wild Kashmiri Iris,
Champion Turkuman Camel-thorn, and that of her son,
American Champion Turkuman Nissim's Laurel, in
the opinion of fellow Afghan breeders will live on in
Afghan pedigrees for ever.

Contents

Illustrations

Introduction

This year, 1970, when I am working on a revised edition (the third) of *The Complete Herbal Book for the Dog*, is, according to the ancient Chinese Calendar, The Year of The Dog (a year which occurs very rarely). This year is distinguished also by a universal interest in natural things, especially food and medicine.

The Complete Herbal Book for the Dog combines all my previous canine herbal works, together with much new material which I have been collecting on my world travels since 1947. I first had published three paperback canine herbals in the mid-nineteen thirties; and it was the first of these books, *The Cure of Canine Distemper*, which established the then absolutely unknown herbal work in the canine world and attracted to herbal medicine many of England's greatest breeders, who, to this day, over thirty years later, are following and advocating herbal treatments as keenly as ever. Two of the first followers in the United States of my herbal writings were Ethelwyn Harrison, of the Shirkarwyn Cockers, Ohio, famous as a spaniel judge, and Sunny Shay, of The Grandeur Afghans, who wrote a new chapter in American canine history in 1959 by winning Best-in-Show at Westminster Championship Show with her famous Champion Shirkhan of Grandeur, who, incidentally, has travelled the whole of America as well as Venezuela, attending shows, and has never been vaccinated against canine distemper or anything else!

My puppy-rearing book, *Puppy Rearing by Natural Methods*, was published in England in 1947 and proved so popular that it went into three editions within the year. It was the first of my canine books to achieve foreign translation, being published by Albert Müller, of Zürich, and my other paperbacks followed there

Introduction

later, in beautifully bound editions. All three books were considered worthy of translation by veterinary professors: *Puppy Rearing*, translated by Dr. Eugene Sieferle, Zürich; *Medicinal Herbs: Their Use in Canine Ailments*, translated by Dr. H. Graf, Veterinary Pharmacology Institute of Zürich University; *Canine Distemper*, translated by F. Granderath, Doctor of Medicine and Veterinary Surgery, Berlin. The puppy-rearing book has achieved seven editions.

My travels in search of authentic and original herbal treatments have been the basis of all my herbal work, and the travels continue. I have covered much of North America and Mexico recently, and Turkey. I agree very much with the opinion of the great herbalist and doctor of medicine of the Middle Ages, Theophrastus Paracelsus Von Hohenheim, usually known as Paracelsus. He urges his students to travel in search of medical knowledge and experience, and he himself travelled in many lands, learning mostly from peasants and wandering gypsies. He, in time, became healer to kings and princes, for with the knowledge that he had acquired he cured diseases that no other doctor was able to cure. Paracelsus taught: 'The knowledge to which we are entitled is not confined within the limits of our own country, and does not run after us, but waits until we go in search of it. No one becomes a master of practical experience in his own house, neither will he find a teacher of the secrets of Nature in the corners of his own room.'

Although the photographs are an important feature of this book, I have had to limit them to about two dozen in order to keep down the cost of my book. I have included cat, goat and bird, because all respond equally well to Natural Rearing and herbal treatments as likewise do bees! I raise bees which are prized for their good health and resistance to disease, and also prized for their rich honey.

One very important illustration I have particulary chosen is a reproduction of a postcard issued by The World Federation for the Protection of Animals, Zürich, Switzerland, because this pleads for the chained dog. I have seen the chained ones everywhere on my travels. In English town yards and on farms, on Spanish and Mexican farms, as protectors of factories and lonely properties in America, and guarding barracks and arms dumps in Israel. In most cases their lot was as described on the 'watchdog' illustration. One day, chaining will be made illegal; certainly it is unnatural.

14

Introduction

Herbal medicine has grown as the herbs themselves, which are spread over the face of the earth, healthful and ineradicable. For this medicine has clean roots, free of all commercial exploitation of animals, and, above all, it is part of Nature's own all-wise teachings.

There are many people to whom the idea of using herbs (which can be bought dried, or otherwise skilfully prepared, by those who cannot gather them wild, as I do) to treat the ailments of their dogs appears nonsensical, or impossible. Yet these books, first published at my own expense because of the prejudices of orthodox veterinary medicine, have sold in their thousands. They have not sold because of any literary merit or appeal to those who buy a herbal book for 'quaint' country lore and 'amusing' extracts from old works; they have sold because every book has meant cures in a widening circle of success, convincing orthodox veterinary surgeons throughout Europe and America.

The letters from dog owners and breeders, which I have found space for in this book, are not included as testimonials for patent medicines; they are the supporting evidence for my unorthodoxy. They mean that these writers, and hundreds more for whom I have no space, who tried my cures with scepticism, have saved their dogs from suffering and death, and have written in gratitude. Spread over a thirty-year period, covering all breeds and representing all classes of dog owners, they are better evidence for the success of my methods than can be shown by many manufacturers of chemicals sold by the shallow magic of advertising.

I would say to all dog owners whose prejudices are aroused by my opinions, my ideas, or even my literary style: Please ignore me. It is not what I think that matters; it is your dog. Give him a chance and try my herbal treatments when science fails; if possible, give him a better chance by trying herbs before it may be too late.

Distemper, hard pad, mange, and many other newer diseases, destroy hundreds of pets and show dogs every year, because the vet called in by the trusting owner frequently says that nothing can be done, for he will not try herbal remedies that have stood the test of countless centuries in many countries. I ask you neither to believe me nor to condemn my treatments until you have tried them. My purpose in writing this book is to save your dog, who should not be denied his chance of Nature's remedies by the prejudices of his owners.

Introduction

Herewith I must register my thanks to the breeders, great and small, who have pioneered my canine herbal treatments throughout the world. To Professor Dr. Edmond Bordeaux Szekely and the late Sir Albert Howard, for their interest and encouragement in the early years. To Richard de la Mare, Chairman of Faber & Faber, my publishers in England, for his endless personal help and encouragement. To the late Arthur Marples, editor of *Our Dogs* journal, England, who described my herbal work as 'important' as long ago as 1935, when it was a tiny and weak seed, and gave me so much space to speak freely for herbs in his important journal. Also to the late Leo C. Wilson, F.Z.S., international judge, journalist, and editor of *Dog World*, England, who constantly supported my work despite the attacks he had to face thereby; to P. R. Moxon, the great gun-dogs expert and author, of *The Shooting Times*, who, calling my herbal book his 'canine Bible', has spread far its teachings; and to P. M. C. Toepoel, international judge, of Holland, for his kind foreword to the Dutch edition of my canine herbal.

Part One

NATURAL PUPPY REARING

1

Diet for Dogs

This chapter is of supreme importance to the book; in comparison, the other chapters become merely supplementary. 'You are what you eat!' was once a maxim of the ancient physicians, although they were not totally correct; for as far as the human being is concerned, what you think also plays an important part in health.

With dogs you can feed good, indifferent, or bad health. It has long been one of my joys of animal rearing by Nature method to watch, day by day, stock growing up in perfect and lasting health, knowing beyond all doubt that on the food that I was giving to them, and the exercise that I was providing for them, day after day, they would increase in health, and they would never—indeed, could not—know disease. Dogs, goats, horses, all have proved the benefits of the natural rearing as opposed to the artificial or scientific.

How different was the case in those kennels in which I spent my early training days as a kennel worker shortly after leaving the veterinary college where I was intending to qualify as a veterinary surgeon, but stayed only a short while (under three years). Both at the university veterinary college and in the various kennels —they included several of England's best-known kennels—I saw much disease. Early puppy losses were calmly accepted as the general rule, and every kennel lived in a superstitious dread of distemper, which amazed me.

It seemed to me so completely wrong, this acceptance of inevitable disease: why should all of the domestic animals, together with human children, be so afflicted with disease, while other creatures—for example, the wild birds—remained almost totally immune? Surely the root cause lay in the hands of man? Man

Diet for Dogs

caused disease, inflicted this unnatural state upon everything which came under his unhappy domination, from animal to plant. I soon began to admire everything that was wild; the shining health of wild ponies and wild deer which I met with in the uninhabited parts of Europe, where I used to stay whenever possible, always inspired me, as did the health of the wild plants in contrast to the cultivated ones. I have never found blight on a wild rose: but just think of, and contrast with, the cultivated roses—which frequently suffer a multitude of diseases. To keep my own life and the life of all animals in my care—dogs, goats, horses—as close as possible to Nature, then became a campaign of paramount importance to me; and the resultant good health of my animals and myself has been sufficient reward for any trouble involved.

That is the first and supreme law of healthful puppy rearing, a natural life and a diet of natural foods. The natural life will be fully dealt with in the chapter on general care of puppies (see page 76); this chapter is primarily concerned with diet.

Canine diet is referred to in Chapter 2 on page 49 and also in that on puppy weaning, but now I should like to deal fully with this subject, keeping in mind always that it rests in the hands of the human owners as to whether an animal is to live its full life span in true and total health, or to be cut off by disease in early infanthood, or to live a miserable life of subhealth.

MEAT FEEDING

The dog is of the family carnivora and he was a flesh-eating beast in his wild state. Well-preserved skeletons of wild or semi-wild dogs show that they were superbly healthy.

Therefore, first and foremost, the dog is a meat eater, its entire anatomy being adapted for a meat diet, from the teeth fashioned for tearing and crushing, the powerful jawbones and muscles, the small, very muscular stomach, the short intestines (to avoid putrefaction of flesh foods), and, above all, the very powerful digestive juices peculiar to the carnivorous animals—digestive juices that can dissolve even lumps of bone. In health, the dog's juices, both of mouth and stomach, are strongly antiseptic, and thus 'high' meat and even flesh from diseased animals—food which would kill a human being in a day—can be eaten without harmful effects. But meat of an unnatural (very inflamed) colour should be avoided.

Diet for Dogs

It generally denotes previous high fever of the animal; dogs usually reject it.

The digestive capacity of the dog is very small when compared, for instance, with that of a goat—an animal of a size similar to that of some of the big-breed adults. The herbivorous animals— horses, cattle, etc.—have enormous capacity for food and can consume many pounds of grain and herbage in a short space of time; whereas the dog, with its small stomach, has room for only very limited quantities of food. Consequently, the general feeding rule for dogs is small amounts of highly concentrated foods, of which raw meat is one of the foremost. Raw meat, fed in lumps, exercises to full capacity both the muscular stomach and the intestines, also the digestive juices, and, of course, utilizes the special teeth and the jaw formation. If other food is substituted, to the extent that such food is fed so likewise there is deterioration of the carnivorous organs of digestion. In view of all this, it is understandable that raw meat should form 75 per cent of the diet of every carnivorous animal.

On the subject of meat feeding, Shikari Man Mahipal Sinha, the chief hunter to the Maharajah of Namli, Central India, sent me an interesting letter. He fully agreed with my findings that a basically flesh diet is the only healthful one for all carnivorous animals, and his hunting hounds were all flesh fed. Only during the very hot seasons it became inadvisable to feed flesh, and the hounds were kept on a light diet of cooked whole-grain cereals, milk products, and similar food. The above findings are quite acceptable to me; I understand well that in countries of extreme climate, where dogs are employed in strenuous work, there are periods of heavy feeding (flesh diet) followed by long intervals of rest, when the dogs are kept on a semi-fasting diet. The Namli hunting hounds are kept on a light cereal diet; while, for instance, the Arctic sleigh dogs receive little food at all during the summer season. When they are retired from work and are turned loose, they have to exist mainly on a diet of raw fish, much of which they must secure for themselves.

Meat is a highly concentrated food; for when the herbivorous animal is in good health its flesh should be made up of the important and highly nutritive vegetable foods on which it has nourished itself; green herbage, whole-grain cereals, sweet brook waters, root vegetables, and silage (such foods are given in natural rearing

21

Diet for Dogs

of cattle, as opposed to the artificial cattle cake, acid-treated straw —even sawdust!—which produce sickly, unhealthy, overfat flesh). Raw flesh contains the cellulose vegetable foods, which cellulose the dog can digest only with difficulty and in very limited quantities in the raw state, turned into protein by herbivorous digestion and now available as muscle, and easily assimilable by the dog. Such meat food has a fair vitamin and mineral content and is absolutely natural food for the dog; just as, to a similar extent, it is unnatural for the human being, to whom flesh food, because of its putrefactive nature, in combination with the human's non-carnivorous bodily structure (his lengthy digestive system), causes an excess of urine with consequential hardening of the human arteries and ligaments, leading to the unnatural onset of early senility. Flesh-eating animals void what they eat in approximately eight hours; whereas human beings require, generally, forty-eight hours and have thirty feet of intestines to pass all food eaten. But there is no space here for reference to the vast subject of human diet. I must refer breeders to the excellent books on the subject by my friend Professor Dr. Edmond Szekely, and published by The Essene School, Tecate, California, U.S.A., and the C. W. Daniel Co. Ltd., Rochford, Ashingdon, Kent, England. But I would like to say here, now, that since human beings (fortunately) are unable to eat meat in its raw state, and therefore must cook all flesh foods, they thereby are losing most of the life-giving properties of that food; for cooking kills both vitamin content and those very valuable and as yet immeasurable cosmic forces, which collect in the flesh of herbivorous animals from the vegetable diet consumed.

Today there is little choice from the town butchers or general markets. The goat flesh and the sheep flesh on which the stalwart hunting hounds of the East are raised, and which are the type of flesh best suited to an animal of the dog's build, are rarely available. The toy breeds would thrive better on a diet of rabbit flesh or of poultry. I would suggest breeders make good use of such flesh foods as the following: breast of mutton (the small bones can also be fed, and are readily digestible by any dog in normal health, i.e. with strong, muscular intestines); sheep heads, including the very nutritious eyes and brain (there is little risk of infection from the parasites that sometimes inhabit the brains of sheep; the good done by such foods offsets any slight risk there may be, since in any case a healthy animal is generally immune to the internal develop-

Diet for Dogs

ment of any parasite—worm or bacteria); ox cheeks, a readily digestible part of the carcass and rich in minerals (sheep heads and ox cheeks can be fed on the bone—the dog will readily tear off all the flesh); and paunches of all animals (the raw, uncleaned paunches of healthy grass-fed animals can be fed with much benefit to all breeds of dogs). I learned this from a gypsy in the Forest of Dean: this man had bred many famous greyhounds, and he told me that such fare was the finest of natural food tonics.

I have fed as he recommended, with great benefit to my dogs. Needless to say, all of the flesh foods given above are to be fed in their raw state only; no cooking of flesh foods can ever be tolerated in natural rearing (or N.R.). Guts of rabbits and hares can also be utilized. Rabbit guts can cause tapeworm, but the tapeworm is short-lived in the truly healthy dog; and in any case an orthodox diet of cooked foods is a far greater cause of long-duration tapeworm. Lewis Godfrey, of the Don Kennels, Hastings, Michigan, U.S.A., writes very sensibly of the feeding of entrails to his borzois. He feeds all types: beef, chicken, fish. He emphasizes the richness of the fat which coats them, and states that most borzois lack fat in the diet. Lack of raw fat is indeed true of the orthodox diet of most breeds. However, only limited amounts should be given.

Finally, how meat should be fed. The foremost law has just been given: *always* raw. Many veterinary surgeons—dominated by Pasteur's unnatural and faulty *germ theory of disease*—advise the sterilizing, by cooking, of all meat fed to the dog. This has also been the official ruling at the British Government dog-training centres (for war dogs), where the consequent health record of many dogs has been unsatisfactory (much loss of young stock from disease, especially distemper, in spite of the distemper vaccination having been rigidly enforced). The main reason why dog owners cook meat is the sheer superstition that such food is made more safe. The theory is as outworn as that of Lister, who poured his ill-famed carbolic-acid disinfectants on to raw wounds in order to kill the 'disease' germs, and who thereby killed off all of the beneficial bacteria which are responsible for tissue healing, and who consequently retarded (sometimes totally so) the healing of most wounds upon which his unnatural treatment was practised.

Destructive measures of any sort will never prove beneficial to life, and the feeding of meat or milk destroyed by being submitted to the forces of heat will only bring positive health degeneration,

23

Diet for Dogs

for nobody can know true health when fed on dead matter; and all cooked foods—with the exception of the naturally tough grains of cereals, which are well used to exposure to the burning heat of the sun's rays in their natural ripening and therefore to some extent resist the destructive forces of fire cooking—are unnatural spoiled substances.

The cooking of meat is more mischievous in its results than the mere killing of the life-forces which are present in all organic substances. Cooking semidigests—artificially—the substance so treated; and in this unnatural breaking-down of the meat tissues, the rightful work of the stomach, intestines, and digestive juices having already been undertaken before the food is fed to the dog, these organs are left improperly exercised; and when this procedure is repeated day after day, it is understandable—it is indeed a law of nature—they will soften and atrophy, so that in time they will be unable to cope with their natural work. Further, the delicate taste buds of the mouth will have become what in medical parlance is known as 'depraved': i.e. an aberration from natural diet; the high-tasting properties of cooked flesh will cause dogs to reject their normal diet of raw flesh for the palate-excitant one of cooked food. Appetite and food preferences, as with man, are no guide to the suitability of foods for the domestic dog. For, resulting from the feeding of unnatural foods for many generations, diet tastes can become perverted.

Now, thousands of dogs—in fact, when pets are taken into the counting, the majority of dogs—are fed habitually on a cooked-foods diet: many are deprived altogether of meat foods; and dogs so fed survive. It is true they are hosts for a multitude of worms, they have unpleasant body smells, have bad breaths, and age rapidly; 70 per cent of them have disordered kidneys by their seventh year, also failing eyesight and hearing; their teeth so filthy with a brown 'fur' deposit that they have to be scraped regularly by a veterinary surgeon. But they survive. How very different is the effect of such diet upon an animal whose ancestors have been reared on a strict raw-foods diet for many generations, and who has been weaned and reared through half of its puppyhood period on the selfsame diet, when it is suddenly placed on foods which are entirely foreign to its system—filthy foods. The harmful effect upon the body, including the nervous system, can well be imagined and understood. Therefore, when you strictly nature-rear any stock,

24

Diet for Dogs

take precautions that those who acquire your animals will continue with the same health diet. I personally, as well as many other breeders, can promptly tell from examination of the teeth, limbs, and eyes whether or not an animal is being naturally reared, and we are seldom mistaken. As many breeders have told me: 'They look so different! They are so vitally alive!' When one meets them in the show ring, the naturally reared stock make the other stock look stiff and aged; it is no wonder that at the present time so many of the c.c. winners at dog shows are N.R. stock, as the photographs in this book will illustrate.

One of the worst faults of cooked flesh and most other cooked foods, especially milk—cooking having changed the nature of the substance—is the after effects when kept for any length of time. This is entirely different from the natural. Raw flesh, when kept for many days, especially during warm weather, becomes 'high' or 'gamey'; it acquires a strong smell; sometimes, also, a grey mould forms; internally, it becomes very tender. It can be fed to any animal with perfect safety, it being quite natural for the dog to partake of flesh in such a state. Indeed, the digging-up and eating of long-buried flesh is one of the delights of the truly healthy dog whose natural instincts have not been spoiled by a cooked-foods diet, for it must always be remembered that *the dog is a natural scavenger* just as much as he is a killer. Very different is cooked meat after storing for many days. This meat turns green in hue and becomes sweaty. To feed 'high' cooked meat is to feed true poison in every sense of the word.

Mr. J. Fairfax-Blakeborough, whose always interesting articles, in, *Dog World* (of England) and elsewhere, which reveal him as being a true student and lover of Nature, upholds my persistent writings on the essential feeding of flesh foods in their raw state. He also makes mention of the old-time greyhound breeders' preference for mutton, this food having always been my own preference for all dogs other than the very big breeds, who can fare quite well on the coarser horse or cow flesh. To quote from Mr. Fairfax-Blakeborough's article in *Dog World*: 'A friend of mine who has somehow managed to keep a considerable number of terriers, hounds and other dogs during the war years, argues in favour of raw-meat feeding. If dogs find a buried sheep they dig it up and eat it, and seem to relish and thrive on such carrion, so that I am not at all sure that this is not *getting very near to Nature*,

Diet for Dogs

upon which man can rarely improve.' (The italicizing is my own—
J. de B. L.) 'Dining the other evening with Mr. D. W. E. Brock, who
has just taken over the amalgamated Cumberland packs, he told me
that he had found feeding raw flesh produced the hardiest and fittest
hounds, that he does not think kennels will ever go back to oatmeal
on the same scale, and although he has had on occasion to boil
flesh to prevent it from becoming tainted, he has often fed hounds
when it was "not all that it should be" without any ill results.' (If
kennel owners would acquire the habit of digging deep pits among
the roots of a shady tree, and placing the meat therein, all the problems of flesh becoming tainted would be overcome, as buried meat
'ripens', it does not taint—J. de B. L.) '. . . Then followed an interesting discussion whether such carcasses could not well be used
in view of the natural habits of the canine species, which preferred
meat which had been buried for some time, and which seemed to
prove by subsequent coat and condition that it suited them.'

*I often feel when thinking back on my canine work, that if I am
able to instil two reforms into the canine world: the fasting of all
dogs in sickness, and the strict feeding of only raw flesh—never
cooked meat in any form—then my years of canine work will not
have been wasted ones.*

The problem of keeping raw meat safe from the ravaging attacks
of blowflies during the spring and summer month, is not an easy
one, especially when large quantities are in use and the kennels are
situated a considerable distance from a meat-supplier. That is one
of the reasons why kennels of few inmates are advocated in preference to over-populated ones.

Fifteen Afghan hounds (including the puppies) was the largest
number of dogs that I ever kept at one time, and that number was
too many. I was able to have raw meat available for them always,
including the hottest months of summer, for I used the ancient
Eastern way of burying the meat in the ground in a shady place.

Buried Meat

The meat must be free from all fly eggs, for otherwise these will
hatch out, even after deep burial, and will spoil the meat. If fly-
blown, *all* the eggs must be scraped off carefully and the cleansed
meat then patted over with a swab of cotton dipped in vinegar.

The pit dug should be a deep one, for sufficient coolness during
hot weather, and the floor should be lined with tree branches or

Diet for Dogs

slabs of stone; tree branches or stone slabs should also be placed over the meat before replacing the soil. These will protect the meat against over-soiling, not that a little soil matters when it is clean. This burying method keeps the meat well and also 'ripens' it. A gypsy told me how his people ripen apples (wild crab apples) by digging pits in the ground, lining the pits with straw, and placing the apples therein. Apples can be kept for months that way. The pit area should be in tree shade preferably, and must be marked with a stout stick, otherwise it may be difficult to find. This may read like a lot of trouble, but far less trouble than washing greasy food dishes and pans, resultant from cooked-meat feeding, and nursing diseased animals also resultant from such feeding.

Stonehenge, the great British canine writer of ancient times, advocated giving raw flesh a coat of whitewash and hanging it in the shade of a tree in order to preserve it. He stated that flesh so treated will keep edible for a month or more. To quote: 'Flesh may be kept for a long time even in summer, by brushing it over with a quick-lime wash, or dusting it with the powder, and then hanging it up in trees with thick foliage. In this way I have kept the shank ends of legs and shoulders good for six weeks in the height of summer and in the winter for three months.'

Small amounts of meat can be placed in brown paper bags or cotton flour bags, the necks tied with string to prevent fly penetration, and hung from a wire coat hanger on a shady tree branch. The wire hook of the hanger will usually deter ants, but if they should defy this, a piece of cloth must be soaked in paraffin daily and wound around the hook base of the hanger. Vinegar can be used on such meat as a mild preservative, using two tablespoons of vinegar to one cupful of cold water. Then wrap the meat around with big, green leaves.

And, after all, there is always refrigeration! If this is on low freezing, little harm will be done to the health properties of the meat. But hard freezing is as destructive as cooking to the health of the meat and to those who consume it. Frozen (iced) food should be used with great caution as it causes ulceration of the digestive track. I have noted the care peasants take to prevent their animals from eating roots and other crops touched by frost. Refrigerated meat must be thawed out and, if necessary, well scalded with hot water.

In the wild, hair and underskin are part of a natural flesh diet

27

Diet for Dogs

and supply essential roughage to exercise the strong muscles of the digestive tract, acting also as a mild laxative. Since in our time the tanner claims animal hides, a little bran should be used instead. Bran supplies roughage and also vitamin B. It has little food value, but it is of a protein nature, although a cereal product. Merely sprinkle a small quantity of bran over the meat feed for each dog; bran ration for an average-sized dog would be about one tablespoon. When bran is unobtainable, a little flaked oats can be used. Oats also are roughage and protein-rich. A small sprinkle will not break the cereal-and-protein-separation rule. When possible, feed meat on the bone in order to encourage the use of the natural canine tearing action. Many of my hounds have swallowed rabbits whole, their strong digestive organs being well able to dissolve and digest the prey, including hair and bones.

Ground-up (minced) meat is especially bad for health as it deprives the dog of jaw and intestinal exercise. Also it often contains too much fat and is harmful, therefore, to health of liver and arteries.

Animals in the wild, after tearing off some outer skin and flesh of their victims, unfailingly show a preference for certain organs of the body: first the intestines, then the eyes. The intestines supply a good source of semi-digested starch and green herbage in the vegetable-eating animals on which the canine races prey usually. (The subject of starch will be fully dealt with subsequently.) The other chosen organs are the eyes, which animals gouge out with great eagerness. (Seagulls, which are partly carnivorous, always greedily seek the eyes of drowned bodies, animal or human.) It is no doubt some minerals salts which attract the carnivorous animals, phosphorus and iodine being present in the eye tissue, normally. Dr. Weston A. Price, writing in a dental journal concerning the Indian tribes of northern Canada, states: '. . . they know that the tissues forming the back part of the eye are good for food. Science has recently demonstrated that the retina of the eyes is one of the rich sources of vitamin A.' The teeth are never acceptable, even as roughage, unless the animal is swallowed whole, in the case of rabbits and other lesser prey, on which the carnivores feed; they are then expelled in the faeces.

RABBITS AND POULTRY. Rabbits and hares are among the best and most natural sources of protein for the dog. Their sharp-splintering bones can be dangerous, especially when cooked. But when the rabbit is eaten by the dog in its natural form—i.e. whole,

Diet for Dogs

including hair, etc.—the hairy skin prevents any danger from bone-splintering and puncturing of the stomach or intestines.

That loathsome man-caused rabbit disease, myxomatosis, so far has not been found harmful to dogs. Some hares have also died from myxomatosis. If any dogs should get the disease they should be treated as described for Distemper and Hard Pad.

A note must be added on the fact that in order to feed rabbits and poultry raw, they should be used fresh, when the flesh is still warm. The flesh of such animals stiffens when cold and becomes rather indigestible.

Therefore, when feeding long-killed shop-bought rabbits, it is advisable to dip the flesh in hot—just off the boil—water and keep submerged for two to three minutes. This will restore the natural elasticity of the flesh without destructive cooking. Some bran or oat flakes should be added as roughage substitute for hair or feathers and to prevent bone-piercing danger.

The same treatment applies to poultry, the flesh needing some quick softening in a little hot water.

LIVER. The dog's natural craving for this organ of the animal body is explained by its high vitamin content and the rich source of natural minerals found in this organ. Liver has long been an accredited cure for anaemia in human beings, but only very recently has it been discovered that there is a unique acid present in liver, and this acid is solely derived from the green 'blood' of leaves; indeed, the acid has been named folic acid, from *folia*—leaf. Common sense would indicate that, in the case of human beings who are well able to assimilate vegetable matter, it would be far more practical to obtain the leaf acid from its source, raw green salads, than indirectly through the liver organ of any animal!

Just as animals seek out the eyes and intestines of their prey, they also seek the liver and the adrenal glands. Indeed, an animal which has not had its natural instincts thwarted and undermined has a very definite plan of action when partaking of the body of its prey. However, the liver is frequently a very unhealthy organ in an unclean animal, as it is the great biochemist of the body, handling many toxic substances, and therefore often overworked. It is one of the first organs to become diseased when the health of the body declines. It can become the storeplace for all manner of body impurities and toxins. In the sheep it can be infected with fluke, a dangerous parasite. Therefore, only feed liver when it is known beyond all doubt that it came from a healthy animal; and, even so, liver is a common cause of diarrhoea in dogs and cats; therefore feed sparingly; not more than twice a week.

TRIPE. This is a suitable food when raw, fresh, and tender. It has to be cut up in quite small pieces. Once frozen or cooked, it becomes indigestible.

CANNED MEAT. This is an unnatural food and causes overeating and bloating. Nature never taught the dog either to cook or to use a can-opener! It is understandable that an amount of chemical preservative is nearly always utilized to keep such food from souring. The food is 'dead' matter in every sense of the word. The spices and other flavouring materials with which it is generally mixed, induce artificial hunger in the dog to which it is fed, and this may damage the stomach lining and the normal balance of the digestive juices. How can any thinking person expect to keep an animal really healthy on preserved food from a tin or bottle? The popularity of such food, supported by large-scale and clever advertising, in my opinion is one reason for the extraordinary increase and variety in canine disease today, when it has become quite usual to feed dogs largely on such totally unnatural fare. Canned meat usually produces over-copious faeces of bad odour.

BONES. When fed raw, they are the canine and feline toothbrush. Through exercise, they also improve jaw structure and promote the length of the jaw. I have always had exceptional foreface on my Afghan hounds, and I know that jaw exercise (plus the feeding of powdered seaweed) has been the reason for this. Soft bones are best for regular use, or flat bones such as ribs, because the hard (marrow-filled) ones are apt to wear down the teeth unduly. Bones which splinter and bones small enough for the dog to swallow whole, as well as poultry and sharp fish bones, should be avoided. Sheep heads, sliced in half, are good and can be fed frequently with the flesh on, for the dog to pick clean. An old-fashioned food for foxhounds is quickly obtained by boiling a whole sheep head with the wool on it and pouring the resultant stock, when tepid, over oatmeal cereal. Personally I do not feed soup of any kind to my dogs or cats; but for those who wish to do so, the foxhound kennel's way is useful. The brains content of sheep heads is very rich in minerals, and dogs will eat it raw.

Diet for Dogs

FISH

Fish is not a recommended canine food. It is too watery and bloodless for the carnivores. However, some breeds of dogs, especially the Portuguese water spaniels, who catch fish for themselves, and some species of Arctic dogs, get almost a mono-diet of fish and flourish on such diet. But they will be obtaining their fish sea- or river-fresh and therefore the flesh is supple and easily digested. The strong, healthy natives of many islands of the South Seas, spear and eat raw, sea-fresh fish. Fish many hours old must be treated the same way as advised for rabbits and poultry, that is, scalded well with hot water to remove the unnatural stiffening of the flesh.

Mackerel and herring are the best fish for canine diet, being extra rich in fats (often lacking in canine diet), nerve vitamin B, and vital minerals. The innards should always be fed, only the heads discarded. A sprinkle of flaked oats is healthful with such rich fish. It can be fed once or twice a week as a change from raw meat. Canned tuna fish is nutritious; its only preservatives are salt and oil.

Lightly steamed white fish, such as cod or plaice, etc., is the ideal 'first' protein for an invalid diet, to be followed by raw meat (see Internal Cleansing Diet Chart, Chapter 5).

GENERAL FEEDING (CEREALS)

Cereal feeding is of far less importance than meat feeding, but it is important enough, for it is on cereals that carnivorous life relies for most of the all-essential minerals as well as the majority of vitamins, including the vital fertility vitamin E, present in the germ of cereals, especially in wheat and maize.

The immense feeding value in cereals can be understood when one stops to think upon the magnificent health of a bull or stallion, raised on a vegetable diet. Dog owners who feed only meat and exclude cereals altogether are making a dietary error, and animals so fed cannot possibly enjoy total health; their diet being one-sided will likewise give one-sided health. Equally bad is the feeding of popular white-flour cereals, for the food value of such is almost nil: all the essential minerals, vitamins, and cosmic forces which

Diet for Dogs

account for the dog's need for cereals are totally lacking in white flour, which merely forms a gluey paste in the stomach, the cause of the prevalent canine gastric disorders and general deficiency diseases, including rickets. It should be remembered that the dog always obtained some semi-digested cereals in his diet. His first action in killing his prey was—and still is—to rip open the abdomen and devour the grains and vegetable matter contained in the intestines of their usually herbivorous prey. That way they would also obtain some barks of trees from the intestines of rabbits or goats, excellent food for dogs.

Such grains, vegetables, herbs, and barks obtained in that way would be semi-digested by the prey before its death, as the vegetable-eating animals chew and salivate, much digestion taking place in the mouth as well as in the intestines; they do not bolt food whole as do the carnivores. Therefore, it is understandable that unlike flesh food, cereal grains fresh from the plant itself cannot be digested by the dog, such food generally passing through the intestines of the dog almost untouched. (It must be mentioned that during the modern world-wide myxomatosis plague, artificially spread by man among the rabbit population, the fox was found to be robbing the wheat when starved of its largely rabbit diet. Intestines of slain foxes were filled with wheat and oats direct from the plants, and the animal avoided starvation on such a diet.)

Some preparation of cereals is therefore required for dogs, and the best method is flaking of the cereal by passing it through heated rollers, as is done in the flour mills. Wheat needs different treatment, and should be ground finely and lightly cooked in order to render it digestible. The flaked cereals should be soaked overnight in cold vegetable stock, plain cold milk, or buttermilk. (Personally, I do not use meat or fish stock for my dogs, as it is apt to sour the cereals and thus likewise sour the intestines.)

Young corn (maize) can be fed raw from the fields when the cobs are young and milky. Merely grate the grains (kernels) finely with a vegetable-shredder, then mix with a little vegetable oil and milk and add a pinch of salt. I feed this often to my Afghan hounds and to my children.

Dog owners can bake their own *wholewheat* dog cakes (soft), using the speedy way of the Bedouin Arabs. Merely mix several pounds of slightly warmed wholewheat flour, using warm water

Diet for Dogs

or buttermilk, honey and molasses (two tablespoons), salt (two teaspoons), added to every quart of water used. Leave in a warm place to rise a little (without yeast). After fifteen minutes, make a hole in the centre of the dough and pour in two dessertspoons of olive oil (or corn oil) to every two pounds of wholewheat flour used. Leave to rise a further thirty minutes, then sprinkle with a little dry flour and form into small flat cakes. Bake on oiled trays in a hot oven for approximately forty minutes. The aim is quick baking to prevent destruction of the vital wheat germ. Solid 'Arabian' cakes result, excellent for teeth and jaw development. My children also flourish on such fare. I do not use *yeast* as, despite the praise given to it by the medical profession, it is an active ferment and can convey the fermentation to the stomach and other organs, causing much internal upset. Professor Edmond Szekeley, author of many books on natural diet and a world-famed authority on diet, warns against the use of yeast. The Bedouins also make *petah*. The flour is then almost raw, merely cooked a few minutes on hot plates.

When in southern Spain I learned to make *toasted* flour, using wholewheat or wholemaize (corn) flour. When made, it is served semi-liquid with cold, raw milk, or made into small balls to eat raw, using tepid water, olive oil, and salt. To toast flour, place in an iron frying-pan $\frac{1}{4}$ lb. flour, spread out well by shaking, then place the pan containing the dry flour over a low flame (preferably using an asbestos mat beneath the pan, but not essential). With the blade of a knife, constantly lift the flour and turn it over, until all deepens into a pale gold (or dark gold, if yellow corn flour is used). The toasting usually takes around five minutes. Shake the pan frequently. When toasted, allow the flour to cool; then store in tins. A hot oven can also be used, after the heat has been turned off. In this method, shake and mix the flour well several times to prevent burning. The famed greyhounds of Seville and Cordoba are given *harina tostada*—and flourish on it.

There is also the *migas* of the Spanish and Portuguese peasants which I learned to make for my children and dogs while in those lands. Into a pan of slightly salted cold water (approximately a quart), toss six 'teeth' cloves of raw garlic and a few sprigs of thyme, sage, or rosemary, one tablespoon olive or corn oil. Then stir in spoonfuls of wholewheat or maize flour, an approximate half pound of flour to a quart of water. Cook slowly and stir well

33

Diet for Dogs

throughout the cooking, which takes approximately fifteen minutes. Then, when thickened, turn heat very low, place lid on pan, and cook slowly for two or three more minutes. When cold, cut into slices and serve. It can be buttered for extra good taste. Chopped herbs such as chives, mint, parsley, etc., can be added when cold. In sunny climates it is helpful to soak the flour in warm water for several hours, placed out in the full sunlight: it will then cook more easily.

* OATS. Flaked, as sold in packets, they are a vital canine food. Being a very good source of iron, they also cleanse the intestines of impurities. They are a proved vital food for stud dogs and brood bitches. It is on oatmeal porridge that the famous collie dogs of Scotland and other hill regions of Great Britain have been reared. These dogs are known for their stamina and resistance to cold and damp. The Border Collie is one of the few natural domestic breeds still unspoiled by man, and its health record is enviable as compared to that of most domestic breeds ill-reared for generations on unnatural foods.

Packet oat flakes are already pre-cooked during the flaking. Do not cook further, merely soak overnight in cold milk, or cold watered milk or cold vegetable soup (nettles and shredded carrot are excellent for this, also potato skins and pea-pods left over from the household kitchen). Add a little salt. 'Milk of oats' is an excellent invalid drink. Merely pour one quart of hot (not boiling) water over a large handful of flaked oats. Allow to stand overnight. Then strain off the liquid 'milk' by pressing this all out from the oats. Reheat to tepid only, then stir in a pinch of salt and one dessert-spoon of honey or maple syrup.

* BARLEY. This is a great aid in dog rearing because of its medicinal properties apart from its considerable food value. It is rich in the antacid magnesium, and is indeed the most alkaline of the cereals. It is an excellent blood cleanser and blood cooler during hot weather. The Arabs choose barley as the principal cereal for their fine Arabian horses and greyhounds (salukis).

The soothing property of barley flour makes it of value also for

* After many years of trying I was, in the early nineteen-sixties, able to supply for followers of Natural Rearing, a complete cereal food of the four cereals, marked*, blended with sea-salt, dried carrots and herbs. Sold as Natural Rearing flakes, the food has enjoyed ten successful years. Available from the same address as Natural Rearing herbs.

Diet for Dogs

external use, and a poultice of barley flour was once a well-known remedy in old English and French homes for treatment of skin ailments. Barley is also a good kidney remedy, and drinks of barley water should be given daily in kidney diseases.

* RYE. This is an excellent cereal as a change from wheat, etc. But the rye used must be whole grain. In its outer coat it contains fluorine, responsible for the formation of good tooth enamel and strong nails. Being low in carbohydrate and fat content, it is a good food to feed to overweight dogs. It is also good for miniature toy breeds, as it keeps them tiny. It is best fed as rye 'wafers', obtainable in packets from food stores.

* CORN (MAIZE). This wonderful cereal, worshipped by the ancient Red Indians and Mexicans, is the only cereal able to sustain life for many months as a sole food. It is usually fed to the dog pre-cooked and flaked. It is then apt to be overeaten and heats the blood unduly. One handful of flaked maize is sufficient daily ration for an average-sized adult dog. The young cobs can be fed raw, merely grated on a vegetable shredder and mixed with milk. The centre core, to which the kernels were attached, is discarded. This cereal, being sun-charged, is a vital one for fertility, being an excellent glandular tonic. It is one of the supreme foods for growing beautiful and abundant hair and strong teeth. Corn *oil* is valuable; several teaspoons can be added to the mixed cereal feed for an average-sized dog. Avoid degerminated corn flours.

RICE. Dogs enjoy an occasional meal of rice, especially when it is enriched with vegetable oils, such as olive or corn, added when the rice is cold, and a raw egg. The natural brown rice from grocers and health foods shops is best, as this cereal, *oryza sativa*, when it is natural 'native' rice, is famous for its health properties, including its ability to cure dysentery. The properties are thiamine, niacin, and iron, and they are lost during the polishing of rice from its natural brown form into unnatural white. If only white rice is obtainable, then add one tablespoon of wheat bran per cupful of rice to restore some vitamin content and roughage.

LINSEED. This is a valuable winter tonic when fed in small quantities along with the other cereal foods. Linseed is rich in minerals, and its valuable oil is very fattening and is a wonderful hair and nerve tonic when used internally—or externally as a hair stimulant and general massage aid. But linseed cake should be avoided, as it is merely the compressed residue of the seed after the valuable oil has been removed by crushing. Linseed must be prepared carefully, for otherwise, owing to its very tough outer coat, it remains entirely inedible and contains a harmful acid. The seed should be soaked in much water for twenty-four hours. Throw away that water. Next day cook slowly for about thirty minutes, stirring repeatedly in order to prevent its adhering to the pan sides and burning. The fluid obtained during the cooking must not be thrown out, for it possesses valuable mineral salts and some oil. It should be used as a base for other soup, reboiling it along with vegetable waste, leaves, onion and potato skins, etc.

PULSES: BEANS, PEAS, LENTILS

These foods, rich in nitrates and fats, are much used in Spain, Mexico, and the Central Americas for cattle dogs, which do well on them. At least such food is whole and has not had germ and outer layers removed in processing, as with most of the cereals.

All should be soaked overnight in cold water, with a pinch of bicarbonate of soda added to reduce the need for lengthy cooking. To cook, place in boiling water and cook rapidly in as little water as possible until soft enough to be digestible. Flavour with a little salt and add some oil when cold. A small quantity of apple or citrus vinegar, one teaspoon to every one and a half pint of water in which the beans are cooked, also lessens the health-destructive cooking time. The Arabian 'hilbeh'—fenugreek seed, merely soak, without soda, and feed raw, one tablespoon per dog; very nutritious.

ROOT VEGETABLES

TURNIPS, parsnips, sweet potatoes (yams), Jerusalem (tuber) artichokes. All are nutritious and rich in vitamins and minerals. They should be either baked in an oven or sliced for quick boiling in a little hot, salted water. They are best when fed mashed into grain cereals. Parsnips and turnips, boiled and spread on to linen cloths when hot, make excellent poultices for swollen limbs, boils, etc. I do not feed common potato; it is too watery for a canine food and also causes stomach gas and colic.

CARROTS. A root vegetable rich in vitamins and minerals (when properly grown by organic methods), they make an excellent supplement for the canine cereal feed and are blood cleansing and

Diet for Dogs

worm removing. Prepare as advised for the other root vegetables. Also feed a little raw, grated. That way carrots are likely to expel worms. Carrots aid formation of good tooth enamel.

MILK FOODS AND HERBS

MILK will be dealt with in some detail in the section on puppy weaning, and therefore will only receive brief mention now. For it must be understood that milk is not a natural food for the dog; the food is natural to human children, whose parents have for centuries kept cattle for the purpose of milk production, and whose anatomy is best suited to a vegetable diet—milk *is* vegetable matter, in liquid form, as produced by the grass- and herb-eating cow or goat. But to the older puppy and to the adult dog, milk is not a natural food, and when taken in excess it will form mucus deposits, which deposits are frequently the root cause of many of the common canine ailments, especially worm infection. Milk should be reserved for the weaning of puppies and the early feeding of weaned stock, especially in the big breeds when much rapid growth must be fostered; for bitches suckling their young; and for treatment of sick or thin animals. The milk-honey diet for sick animals simply cannot be improved on, and for that reason alone, no person should attempt puppy rearing who is unable to ensure supplies of fresh raw milk at all times. Needless to say, just as it is essential to ensure that cereal foods are obtained from healthy grain, so likewise milk must be of a high health standard, obtained from healthy cows or goats. Disease can be fed to puppies through unclean and unhealthy milk, just as it can through rodent-tainted grain. Care must always be taken to ensure that only healthy foods are fed to all animals on all occasions. I have usually kept my own goats when rearing many young puppies.

BUTTERMILK. This excellent food is an acquired taste in dogs and they should be given it from early puppyhood. Similar to whole, sour 'clabbered' milk, it has worm-removing properties. It is also very blood cooling. It makes a perfect biscuit base, with wholewheat flour mixed purely with buttermilk instead of the plain water usually used.

The secret of making good clabbered milk—and therefore buttermilk—is to keep the milk aerated during the making. The milk should stand in a warm place, or in sunlight, and be topped with thin paper or cotton to keep out flies or dust. Do not sunheat above tepid. The standing milk should be stirred briskly with a fork, morning, midday, and night.

BUTTER. This being an unnatural food, it should be used very sparingly, as it is apt to cause liver trouble in dogs and cats, despite their enjoyment of this food. It can be spread lightly on whole wheat or whole rye bread, and in this way helps to encourage appetite in poor eaters.

CHEESE. Fresh white cheese or cottage cheese is a good food which most dogs, and some cats, enjoy. Solid yellow cheese is indigestible.

HERBS. Most herbs play a very small part in canine diet, although a remarkably important part in canine medicine. The dog is no true vegetable eater, taking only what it gets from the contents of the intestines of the prey which it kills, and in very limited amounts direct from various grasses, berries, and mosses, which it seeks out for itself. Many dogs have completely lost their natural instincts for the seeking-out of herbs; only for that admirable, intestinal cleansing herb, couch grass,[1] do dogs seem to have retained their herb-eating instinct, and even this instinct is often thwarted by their owners, who drag their dogs away from the grass because they do not like its making their dogs vomit up bile, which is the sole purpose, apart from its laxative properties, for which the dog eats couch grass! Modern veterinary surgeons have also been known to advise clients to keep their dogs away from couch grass because it will cause them to vomit and have loose bowels.

WATER

Nearly three-quarters of a dog's body consists of water, and the dog parts with a large amount of this daily via the lungs and urinary organs. Loss of urine is especially heavy after active exercise. Therefore, for health maintenance there must be a constant renewal of the water content of the body by regular intake of this highly important fluid. The dog, especially when sick, can exist for days and weeks solely on water, whereas in general he could not live for more than a limited number of days without intake of water, though there have been exceptions to this fact in the case

[1] *Agropyrum repens.*

Diet for Dogs

of dogs lost down badger holes, old mines, etc., which have survived for weeks even without water.

The water, which the dog replaces daily, must be pure and natural for total health. In the past, when purchasing Afghan hounds to establish my own Turkuman strain, one of my first considerations was the water supply of the kennel that I was visiting. Therefore, I always sought stock from country kennels where there was good water. A famous race-horse breeder once told me that he would not consider land for his mares and foals where there was not a running stream of spring-fed water. He wanted strong bones for the legs of his race-horses, and without good water he could not achieve this.

In our modern civilized life it becomes increasingly impossible to avoid having chlorine and fluorine in our tap water. When I have met with very heavy chemical treatment of water during my travels, I have gone to the expense of purchasing bottled spring water for my children and animals rather than poison their blood with unnatural chemicals.

Drinking-water, put out for dogs, should be changed twice daily. Water-dishes or troughs should be placed in shady places. Collect all possible rain-water so long as this has not fallen through factory- or chimney-polluted air; i.e. so long as it is clean rain-water.

Do not allow drinking immediately after meals, for this washes down the food in a semi-digested state into the lower intestines, causing indigestion and bloating. Puppies require water from an early age. They are thirsty for water long before weaning; they therefore should be provided with shallow dishes of water as soon as their eyes have opened.

MISCELLANEOUS CANINE FOODS

HONEY. I believe I could not successfully rear domestic dogs without this remarkable antiseptic food. It is of course not a normal item of diet for the carnivores, but the lion enjoys honey, and it is considered a staple food of the vegetarian bear, one of the strongest of the wild animals. Honey is the greatest of the natural energizers, a nerve tonic and a supreme heart tonic, indeed it is the only known heart stimulant which is not a drug. Predigested by its makers, the bees, it is absorbed immediately into the bloodstream.

Diet for Dogs

A diet of milk and honey only, can sustain life for months in human animals.

In the famous Frauenfelden Home in Switzerland, sickly infants are placed on a prolonged diet of milk and honey, usually for many weeks, with remarkably good results. The mother of Hillary, the New Zealand beekeeper whose extraordinary stamina enabled him to achieve the first ascent of Mount Everest, together with Sherpa Tensing, in 1953, declared that her son's exceptional strength is much due to the big amounts of honey on which he was reared. The purity of all honey used cannot be over-emphasized. In Europe synthetic honey is a popular article; it has none of the good properties of bee honey and is also bad for the teeth. Purchase honey preferably direct from beekeepers or from health foods stores, and get a guarantee that the honey has not come from areas where fruit trees or plants are sprayed with poisonous insecticides. Also the honey should not be filtered or heat treated, the latter is often done to commercial honey to facilitate the easy pouring of honey into small jars. Therefore it is often best to buy honey in bulk in large cans or jars to safeguard against heat treatment, which destroys 50 per cent of the natural health properties of honey.

In Galilee, Israel, just as I provide medicinal herbs for my goats, dogs, and my own family, I grow a herb garden of special bee herbs. The bees themselves are natural herbalists, and will gorge themselves on bitter rue or pungent lavender and rosemary in preference to garden roses and other merely ornamental flowers (whereas they seek out the wild roses very keenly). The honey provided from the herb garden is naturally very healthful, and buyers come for it from most distant places, and the bees themselves enjoy excellent health and possess complete resistance to the many diseases afflicting the local white-sugar-fed bees.

Feed honey to puppies with their milk meal, and to sick dogs either in their water, if they will take it, or in balls of thick honey pushed down their throats. Honey can also be used externally for treatment of burns (see Scalds, Chapter 6).

EGGS. Eggs from hens, ducks, or turtles are a rich source of mineral salts and vitamins. The shells given in small amounts, pounded into powder by means of a flat stone, are a good form of giving natural calcium to the dog and are a fine aid to the building of well-textured bone. Eggshell is rather insoluble, but the strong

40

Diet for Dogs

digestive juices of the *healthy* dog can cope with it. Breeders, on my recommendation, have been using this natural bone-building aid for many years now and are enthusiastic about the results obtained. Eggs, because of their richness, should only be given in limited quantities. Eggs must be fresh, as staleness renders them indigestible. They should be fed raw, as cooking causes them to adhere to the digestive tract. Feed one egg on alternate days per week to adult dogs and likewise to puppies. Eggs are quite a natural food to the dog, for dogs will seek out and eat the eggs of sea-birds and other birds, such as game-birds, which lay their eggs upon the ground. Eggs are a very *unsuitable* food for sick animals because of their highly fermentative properties. During the heat of fever, for instance, they rapidly poison the body instead of strengthening it. Egg-and-milk has long been the most misguided of the orthodox medical recommended invalid foods; the giving of such food has done about as much to spoil cures by orthodox treatment as has the popular use of the destructive sulphonamide group of drugs.

SEAWEED. Seaweed could be classified with the herbs, but its special properties are so important to canine health that it is being given a separate mention. Seaweed is without equal as a source of natural iodine, concerning which substance Lillian R. Carque, Sc.D., writing in an American journal, states: 'Iodine is highly desirable for pregnant mothers. It is especially needed at the age of adolescence for the development of the reproductive organs, particularly in the female in whom the change-over takes place more rapidly than in the male. Adequate iodine also insures luxuriant hair and skin health; lack gives rise to a very dry skin and loss of hair. Increased iodine intake permits better digestion and assimilation of fatty elements in foods. Organic iodine—the only kind the thyroid gland can appropriate—causes better retention and utilization of calcium and phosphorus; lesser degrees of thyroid deficiency produce bone changes analogous to that of rickets. It is very essential, too, in combating disease germs and their poisonous excretions. The secretions of the thyroid gland are definitely germicidal. Organic iodine raises the red blood-cell count and has a direct influence on the formation of red blood corpuscles. Ages ago Greek gladiators used seaweed as part of their diet. Certain tribes of American Indians were known to make annual trips to the coast to obtain seaweed, doubtless because they ap-

Diet for Dogs

preciated the therapeutic value in arresting disease. Seaweed, a natural sea food, contains no drug principle or stimulant, and is of far greater value in mineral and vitamin content than is much earth-grown produce raised on impoverished soil.'

Seaweed is not an unnatural food for dogs. They would get this from the intestinal contents of herbivorous animals who will eat it in small amounts. As seaweed gives dark pigment to eyes, nose, and claws, the use of seaweed is much acclaimed in the canine world. But no doubt its true fame is due to its powers to stimulate hair growth; and through being a glandular tonic, it also stimulates general forward and stalwart body development and promotes strong bones. I am pleased to have been responsible for introducing and popularizing this wonderful product of Nature among dog breeders throughout the world. I have pioneered this also for cattle, goats, sheep, poultry, and racing pigeons. I first introduced seaweed to the veterinary world when a student in the early 1930s; it was scorned then; now it is in popular use.

COD AND HALIBUT LIVER OIL. This is a further food of value in puppy rearing, especially in sunless climates during the winter months. The main value of these fish oils is their power to combat rickets, and in this they are superior to any other fats, including butterfat. Cod and halibut obtain their rich oils indirectly from seaweeds and one-celled algae. Care should be taken to ensure that the oils are raw and unrefined. Heat treatment is sometimes used and the health of the oil is thereby lost. Use fish oils sparingly, for if used in excess they will sour the intestines. One small teaspoon daily during the winter months is sufficient for an average breed puppy. Do not give during hot weather. Halibut oil is milder than cod, but as it spoils easily, it is best given in capsule form. Both oils should be kept away from strong light and stored in dark-glass bottles. Avocado pear, raw mashed, gives a vital oil.

Final Notes

Dogs should never have their natural instincts thwarted in the matter of diet. They should not be prevented from eating the droppings from grass-fed cattle and horses, from which they can get many vital elements derived from the herbage on which the animals have grazed and in a form easily assimilated by the dog. Likewise, puppies should not be prevented from eating earth. This removes intestinal impurities and worms in the same way as couch-

Diet for Dogs

grass eating, which, as already stated, likewise should be encouraged. Only eating of its own faeces is a depraved habit and should be checked at once.

To complete this chapter, I am giving in detail the Natural Rearing Puppy and Adult Diet Charts, which charts, when they are in *proper* daily use, have banished all disease from dogs. This has been well proved during the past thirty years by kennels in all parts of the world. Adequate exercise and hygienic kennelling are also of importance to achieve this total health. When dog owners have obtained this health among their own dogs, it is hoped they will extend their knowledge to the other animals, cattle, horses, poultry, and so forth, and, of greater importance, to the rearing of their children, who, too, require a basic diet of uncooked natural foods and freedom from the use of chemical medicines and vaccines.

But before giving the chart, I want to mention a subject which so often reaches me: Can dogs be reared on a vegetarian diet? Yes, they can be so reared. But as I am writing this book on natural rearing, I do not want to deal with the unnatural here. A vegetarian diet of whole (mostly raw) foods, giving eggs, cheese, and milk for protein, can keep a dog in good health, but such diet is far more difficult to feed successfully than the natural carnivorous one. However, there are many vegetarian dog owners who are loath to feed meat, and for this reason the London Vegetarian Society asked me, in 1953, to write an article on 'Vegetarian Diet for Dogs and Cats' for their journal—*The Vegetarian News*. The article aroused much interest, and was therefore later issued as a leaflet by the London Vegetarian Society. It is still in print.

NATURAL REARING PUPPY DIET CHART

Puppies reared according to the laws of Nature are always far superior in every way to stock incorrectly reared on the usual unnatural canine diets, and have been found to possess an extraordinary resistance to all disease. Natural Rearing gives exceptionally strong bone, dense body hair, heavy muscle in place of fat, and always sound nerves. The usual puppy ailments do not occur when natural rearing is strictly followed. The four main rules of natural rearing are: (1) correct natural diet of raw foods; (2) abundant sunlight and fresh air; (3) at least two hours' exercise daily (including plenty of running exercise); (4) hygienic kennelling,

43

Diet for Dogs

with use of earth and grass runs to give contact with the vital radiations of the earth. No concrete runs should be used. But the old-fashioned brick or cobblestones, with good drainage provided, can be utilized on very damp land; gravel, likewise, can be used.

Natural Rearing Diet (*from weaning to four months*)

For average breed puppy. For big breeds and toy breeds, increase or decrease accordingly. No puppy should be given other than milk foods before four weeks of age. Finely shredded raw meat can then be given if desired. It is impossible to give exact quantities. All puppies of all breeds differ in appetite capacity. Never give hot food; blood-heat (tepid) or cold is natural. Hot food damages the stomach and intestines and can cause cancer. Animals usually, wisely, refuse to touch hot food.

8 a.m. Fluid meal of raw milk (cow or goat), not dried or canned milk, strengthened with honey and tree barks blend.[1] *Less than ½ pint.*

12 noon. Whole-grain flaked porridge oats, wheat, barley, or rye, or mixed flakes, soaked overnight in cold milk (sour milk is excellent for this), and a few finely chopped raisins, a teaspoonful of flaked margarine. Alternatively, the cereal flakes can be soaked in cabbage or nettle water. Barley, being the most digestible of the cereals, should be used for weaning if available. A perfect cereal meal for growing puppies is two parts barley flakes to one part oat flakes (such as sold in packets for porridge making), soaked in fresh cold milk. A dessertspoon or so of raw cornflour can be added. *Use one large handful of flaked cereal or cereals.* With this meal two or three slices of stale wholewheat bread should be given. When biscuits or meal are preferred, use only chemical-free, farmhouse type of 'health' biscuit, a blend of true wholegrain cereals. If it is desired to feed fruit to the puppy—and finely grated apple is a healthful food—it should be mixed in with flaked cereals and milk.

4 p.m. Meat: approximately two ounces raw, shredded (cow or horse flesh, or breast of mutton—the soft mutton bones may be given). Meat should never be minced, the powerful stomach muscles must be used for meat digestion; after ten weeks of age, meat should be given in pieces about the size of a 5p piece, increasing in

[1] A blend of nutritious barks of trees; my own formula. See Appendix at end of book, page 198.

44

Diet for Dogs

size to pieces as large as a hen's egg after four months. Raw, finely cut herrings sprinkled with flaked oats can be fed once or twice weekly as a change from meat. Scald the fish well to soften it before cutting.

8 p.m. (main meal) Meat: approximately two ounces (as above).

Plus one teaspoonful wheat germ (such as Bemax, Froment, etc.), and equal amount of bran for extra roughage. When bran is not available, a sprinkle of flaked oats can be used.

Plus one teaspoonful cod-liver oil (in winter), olive oil (in summer).

Plus a sprinkle of seaweed powder (rich in natural minerals, especially iodine[1]), promotes dense body hair, strengthens nerves.

Plus one teaspoonful raw green leaves: dandelion, or parsley, or mint, or watercress, or green celery leaves; a mixture of several is good. The leaves must be very finely chopped with a sharp knife, almost to a pulp, as dogs have difficulty in cellulose digestion. The daily ration of green food is essential to health. Raw chopped onion, one teaspoonful, is also excellent, especially when worms or skin disorders are present. Two or three herbal antiseptic tablets, such herbs as garlic, rue, eucalyptus, etc., are recommended several days weekly. Raw eggs on meat occasionally, or raw eggs can be given on the cereal food. It may be necessary to make an incision with a knife on the meat, to prevent the dog from shaking off the supplements, which should be rubbed in. Or use a sprinkle of cold water to make the supplements adhere.

Give large raw bones to gnaw, several times weekly.

Allow plenty of drinking-water, during weaning included, but do not allow drinking soon after meals (cause of gastritis).

After four months, omit the 8 a.m. feeding, and feed only at 12 noon, 4 p.m., and 8 p.m. The cereal allowance should be increased to fully satisfy appetite, the meat to eight ounces or more, and the raw vegetable to one dessertspoon. After seven months, meals should be reduced to two: cereal at midday; meat in the evening, sufficient food being given each meal to satisfy.

Note. Every puppy, from weaning onward, should rest and cleanse its internal organs frequently by fasts on plain water only. A puppy should never be coaxed or tempted to eat. If food is not

[1] See Appendix at end of book, page 198.

Diet for Dogs

eaten rapidly the puppy should be fasted for from twelve to twenty-four hours. Every puppy over four months old should have a half-day fast one day per week (suggested every Sunday); a whole-day fast one day per month. Every adult a weekly one-day fast.

Do not prevent puppies from eating earth or excreta from grass-fed cattle, etc., as this is natural to carnivores. Also encourage them to eat grass.

Important. Throughout this scientific diet, meat and starch foods should not be mixed up at the same meal. They are incompatible and cause scouring, with the resultant indigestion, which is the root of hysteria, gastritis, worms, and other disorders. The only exception is the sprinkle of flaked oats (a protein-rich cereal) to supply extra roughage if bran is not available, or a hard-baked wholewheat crust or biscuit as a finish to promote saliva flow. Also plain milk should not be given in large amounts; it should be fortified with honey or thickened with tree bark flour or whole-grain cereals, thus overcoming the tendency to create mucus. Precautions should be taken against the feeding of soured foods (cereals) during hot weather. Sour food can cause serious intestinal illness. Cooked meat also sours, whereas raw meat only ripens.

The diet given herewith is for show stock and can be simplified for everyday use.

Further Note. The quantities given are for average puppies; larger breed puppies require far greater quantities of food, according to size.

So many people write me for details of correct amounts to give puppies. I have always declined to supply such information, for so much is dependent upon so many variable factors. Breed, build of puppy, quality of food, amount of exercise being given, even the temperament of the puppy in question. Also, it must be understood that growing stock needs more daily food than adult. However, for those persons insistent on feeding by weighed-out amounts, I think that 'Stonehenge's' observations are the soundest that I have yet met with in any canine book. 'The quantity by weight which is received by the growing puppy is from one-twelfth to one-twentieth of the weight of its body, varying with the rapidity of growth and a good deal with the breed also. Thus a twelve-pound dog will take from five-eighths of a pound to a pound of food, and a twenty-six pound dog from two to three pounds. When they arrive at full growth, more than the smaller of these weights is very seldom

46

Diet for Dogs

wanted, and it may be taken as the average lot of food of this kind for all dogs in tolerably active exercise.' ('Stonehenge' advocates a raw flesh and cooked cereal diet for dog-rearing.) However, I think that a dog should be allowed to eat to capacity on plain whole-grain cereals, only controlling the amount of meat. A dog could well overeat on meat, but is unlikely to do so on plain cereals.

Another simple method of calculation is based on the ancient Arab teaching that the human body requires no more than two to three pounds of food per day for health. This basic amount can be reduced according to the size of the dog in question, though remembering that the dog takes more active exercise, thus using up more food, and it was on this teaching that I based the food needs of my Afghan hounds.

One final comment applicable to all puppies is: give puppies as much of natural foods as they will eat up keenly without their stomachs becoming distended after eating.

SPECIMEN DIET FOR AN AVERAGE-SIZE ADULT DOG

Midday. 100 per cent flaked whole-grain wheat, rye, or barley, softened with either raw milk or vegetable juice. I have made available a 4-cereals flakes meal, with herbs, popular with all dogs. Sour milk is excellent for this. Wholewheat, rye, or corn bread, or biscuits of same, also (uncooked) whole-maize flour, can be added to this meal. Also raw eggs can be mixed into the cereal, approximately four times per week. Likewise, some corn, olive, or sunflower oil, one dessertspoon for an average-size dog; use far less if the dog is fat.

Note: No adult dog should be fed before midday; the hours from midnight to midday are strongly eliminative ones. In-between-meal scraps are harmful. However, hunting breeds of greyhound build, with small stomachs, often want an early-morning meal instead of at midday.

Evening (main feed): Meat, raw, in large pieces, never minced. Very hard frozen meat is as harmful as cooked meat. A small quantity of fat should be included.

Plus one teaspoon wheat-germ flakes.

Plus one teaspoon cod-liver oil (winter).

47

Diet for Dogs

Plus seaweed powder.

Plus one heaped dessertspoon very finely chopped raw green herb, such as parsley, watercress, dandelion. The inclusion of the herb is important. Also grated raw carrot can be added.

Plus several dessertspoons of bran or flaked oats to replace lost roughage of the skin and hair.

When bones are given, they should be raw and fed after the meat. They should not be given on an empty stomach.

In-whelp bitches, nursing bitches, and invalid adults, are permitted an early-morning meal of milk and honey; a dessertspoon of bran can be added to prevent mucus formation; also tree-bark flour to be added. When available, grapes or apples, pressed through cheese-cloth or through strong muslin, make a good addition to this morning drink.

All the carnivorous animals need one meatless day per week and one day on fluids only, i.e. five days only of meat feeding. No wild dog would be able to kill prey every day of every week. Appreciating this fact, most of the zoos of the world fast the carnivores—lions, tigers, wolves—one day each week.

For the natural-rearing diet it is recommended there be one meatless day per week, using instead milk, eggs, white cheese with cereal. One fast day should follow this, giving fluids only and a laxative the same night, also herbal pills the next morning. This simple Nature treatment wards off disease toxins, rests the kidneys, which are always overworked on a meat diet, and rejuvenates the dog. Hungry dogs can be given a little honey in their water at meal times, or very watery diluted milk, or water from flaked oats or barley, obtained from pouring hot water over the flakes and soaking them overnight.

Note. An increasing demand in England, America and Canada for natural, whole-grain cereals has made such products as wheat, barley, rye, corn, etc. available in most towns, at many co-operative stores, health foods stores, etc. Many mills supply direct by mail. Firms mailing whole-grain natural cereals are: N.R. Products, England (Old Smithy, Ibsley, Ringwood, Hants) and in U.S.A.: Walnut Acres, Penns Creek, Pennsylvania, and The Great Valley Mills, Kellers Church, Bucks County, Pennsylvania. And there are others. Send to them for their lists.

2

Care of the In-whelp Bitch

My thirty years and more of veterinary medicine work have revealed to me the appalling amount of canine disease prevalent in all parts of the world. Nearly 50 per cent of such disease is hereditary and will require drastic and long-term measures to wholly breed-out from the various strains in which it is manifest. But the other 50 per cent is readily preventable and curable by promptly and wholeheartedly adopting natural rearing (N.R.) rules. The dog is a most simple animal to keep in good health. It has not the complicated digestive system of the human being, for instance, which makes health maintenance or disease cure such a far more involved and long-term business; any child can keep a dog in great health; and yet—because unnatural rearing methods are the rule—the amount of canine disease prevalent in the civilized world today is a horrible thought. To comprehend present-day canine disease, one has only to read through modern veterinary medical textbooks and to study the long lists of ailments which afflict a species of animal, whose anatomy and way of life should by rights enable it to be the healthiest of all domestic animals. Such unpleasant reading must give one reason for thought.

I have written the puppy-rearing section to ensure that all puppies should be given the chance of enjoying their rightful inheritance of good health. When all puppies are reared by such methods, canine disease will positively disappear within a very few generations of N.R. stock. Such has been my own experience, and the experience of leading breeders in England and overseas. The words of Mrs. Wingfield Digby—pioneer Keeshond breeder and owner of the famous Van Zaadam Keeshonds in England—are apt. Writing of N.R. stock, she says: 'Never before have I seen such forward and intelligent puppies. It is as if they felt extra well.'

Care of the In-whelp Bitch

The care of the in-whelp bitch is almost totally neglected in most dog-breeding establishments. The bitch is merely mated and then expected to produce her litter at the end of the nine-weeks' period; no changes in diet or general treatment have been followed at all. In the rare cases when the in-whelp bitch is singled out for special attention, the treatment is generally of a most unnatural nature. There is usually overfeeding, resulting in heavy, inactive puppies, which cause whelping difficulties. Dosage with chemical calcium is supposed to 'grow' strong bone, but in actual fact acts as a kidney irritant and causes unnatural brittleness of the bony structure of the body (also causes rigidity of the bone parts of the litter in embryo, thus making further whelping difficulties). Such neglect of the in-whelp bitch is remarkable when it must be appreciated that the health of the forthcoming litter is much affected by the dam throughout the nine-weeks' in-whelp period. In actual fact, the health of a litter of puppies is 50 per cent dependent on prenatal care and diet.

The Arabs say, concerning their famous Arabian horses, that the stallion gives type to the foals, the mare gives *health*. They pay endless attention to the health of their brood mares. The same care is necessary for the brood bitch, from puppyhood, if she is to produce, when adult, a litter truly healthy and truly capable of improving the health standard of the breed.

Dr. G. T. Wrench, in his important book concerning that natural-living race of people, the Hunza tribe of the Indian mountains, goes even further than my statement concerning the effect of prenatal health on the offspring. He states: 'Unless the mother is healthy and carries healthy blood to her conception, the wholeness of health cannot be attained.' And yet how many bitches are mated year after year when in a state of actual disease: sufferers of skin diseases, kidney diseases, obesity, glandular ailments, and many other sub-health conditions? No wonder that such bitches prove barren, or whelp litters which fade away at birth or are carried off by one or another of the so-called epidemic diseases shortly after weaning. Or if litters bred from unhealthy stock do survive, such stock is malformed with 'shelly' bone and sparse hair, or very subject to worm infestation, or are constant sufferers from one or more of the canine ailments which have long been looked upon as being the normal lot of the canine race.

Appreciating that good bone formation, nerve structure, and

Care of the In-whelp Bitch

hair growth are dependent upon the blood of the dam during the all-important nine weeks of growth in the womb, it is understandable that in any book concerned with puppy rearing, a chapter on care of the in-whelp bitch is essential.

As for the stud dog, good health should again be an essential when making a choice of sire, for through the stud dog, just as with the brood bitch, hereditary ailments can enter and dominate the future lives of the unborn puppies. The mange-type of skin disease prevalent in many strains of chows and dachshunds; chorea in collies and terriers; kidney disease in Scottish terriers; hind-quarters paralysis in Dachshunds and Pekinese; hip disease (hip dysplasia) in Alsatians, Labradors, and Samoyeds; slipped stifle joint in King Charles spaniels and Poodles; epileptic fits in Kerry Blues; deafness in Bull Terriers—these are but a few examples to be found of hereditary diseases in the hitherto healthy canine race; and perhaps the miniature and toy poodles are the worst of all examples of man's unnatural rearing methods, suffering as they do from such inherited ailments as toothlessness, deformed inner ears, and blindness. Then there is among many breeds general epilepsy, chronic skin diseases, heart diseases, diabetes, and so on, all greatly established by vaccinations from stock made artificially diseased in laboratories. Such ailments can now be bred out only with infinite patience and trouble.

As Miss Peggy E. Brown, of Harrogate, who studied agriculture at Reading University, writes: 'Without a doubt it is this everlasting breeding for show points at the expense of all else that is the cause of all the degeneration in canine health. If the things that matter, principally good health, are never bred for, they are *bound* to get lost. It only needs one champion dog to be popular at stud and yet suffering with some serious hereditary ailment, and in no time it will spread right through a breed. Just look how wonderful are the Border Collies—bred for stamina, intelligence, etc., yet never for looks to a Show Standard, nor are they inoculated; yet, despite no Show Standard, they are easily recognizable as a breed, in type. *They* are not wiped out by modern diseases, and they get the roughest, but reasonably nourishing, food, from poultry and pig meal to milk. On raw meat they would become superb. Nothing beyond their reach.'

These collies do get a limited amount of meat at certain seasons, dead lambs, carcasses of dead sheep, also entrails of rabbits. Some

51

Care of the In-whelp Bitch

farmers have a superstitious belief against feeding meat to collies in case they turn 'killers'. But I have been much with Border Collies and have seen them dig up and eat or take from rivers sheep carcasses.

It is a logical consideration, therefore, that the health of a stud dog should be carefully considered when making a selection for breeding; it is of equal importance (of greater importance in my opinion) with show points. Anyway, show merit is largely dependent on good bone formation, hair growth, true movement; all of which are, in turn, largely dependent on sound health. In most breeds (the dog being a carnivorous animal) good strong jaw formation is a desirable show point; growth of jaw is largely determined by good rearing.

In addition to ensuring that a bitch is in the highest possible state of health at the time of mating, the period of the year at which the litter will be born should also be taken into consideration. Spring litters are natural, winter litters unnatural. It is noticeable that newly imported breeds, which have come from lands where they have been allowed to lead a natural, often semi-wild, life, seldom come on heat more than once a year. The females of that hardy wild animal, the jackal, closely related to the dog family (indeed they will mate with dogs), come into season only once a year. They mate for life and remain entirely loyal to one mate. In dog-breeding, bitches should be allowed to mate with dogs for which they show preference. They should never be forced to mate with a disliked dog merely because that dog has good blood lines. Menstruation is often a partial cleansing of the body. The reproductive organs are areas of the body which frequently become very toxin-laden in wrongly reared animals. The on-heat period of a healthy bitch is very short, and there is no evil-smelling discharge whatsoever. In such cases it is purely an outflow of the organs of reproduction in preparation for mating and subsequent birth, there is no cleansing process at all.

Horse breeders wisely place a far higher value on spring-born foals. It is the opinion in the horse world that winter-born foals never attain the stamina of the spring-born.

The milk-feeding question here plays a part. In the spring when cattle are grazing on the new grass, the milk is far better in every way than winter milk. Indeed, winter milk from cows or goats is not a suitable puppy weaning food at all.

52

Care of the In-whelp Bitch

DIET FOR THE IN-WHELP BITCH

The rule of paramount importance in diet for the in-whelp bitch is, of course, feed *raw* foods. The previous chapter described how cooking causes general deterioration of the entire digestive system, from the teeth to the lowermost region of the bowels. Cooked food clogs around the teeth and causes dental decay; also weakness of jaw formation, owing to the bones and muscles of the jaws being insufficiently exercised through the feeding of heat-softened pappy food. The digestive juices are weakened, because cooked food is semi-digested in the process of cooking, and therefore the powerful digestive juices, natural to the dog, are no longer fully required or utilized. The powerful muscles of stomach and intestines, with which the carnivorous races are so well supplied (the digestive juices and intestinal muscles can break down and partially dissolve such hard substances as lumps of bone, skin and hair, pieces of gristle, and so on), in their turn weaken and diminish, they—as with the digestive juices—being deprived of their rightful work, and being insufficiently utilized—just as with an injured limb kept in splints for a lengthy time—become flabby and eventually shrivel. Therefore, for the unborn litter to be properly nourished, the bitch's diet must be mainly raw foods, only a little semi-cooked cereal food being the exception to the rule. Often around the fourth week the bitch will refuse her food and give herself a voluntary fast. This is very frequent and is due to digestive disturbances caused by her condition. She should never be coaxed to eat at such times. At the most she should be offered a raw milk-honey diet. Normal appetite will soon return, and the bitch is generally found to have developed an increased appetite.

It will soon be found that a healthy bitch requires far less food than an unhealthy one. When I think back on the enormous quantities of food that I used to feed my dogs when I was a schoolgirl and university student, and generally I had two or three dogs in my care, I am always left amazed at the recollection. The diet for my borzoi dog, for instance, used to be almost a bucketful of soaked white houndmeal, with lumps of cooked meat supplied with it. The dog used to eat this vast daily feed, but he never fattened and was always ailing with eczema and kindred diseases—and no wonder! My Afghan hounds have attained great height and condition on a

53

general daily ration of 1¼ lb. of raw meat and ½ lb. of whole-grain cereal. Actually, the Essenes, that great sect of Eastern people, unsurpassed doctors, used to rule that no adult human being should consume more than 2 lb. of food daily, for true health. This fact makes one wonder, when the huge quantities of food which breeders give daily to their dogs are taken into consideration. The real solution is that healthy bodies utilize every particle of food fed to them, whereas unhealthy bodies in the main allow most of the food fed to them to pass through the intestines only semi-digested, and therefore twice the normal quantities of food have to be fed to the unhealthy animals in order to prevent excessive thinness and other subnormal health conditions resulting from underfeeding.

A great mistake is made when double-ration feeding of the in-whelp bitch is practised, the idea behind such feeding being that the unborn and rapidly developing litter must be well and sufficiently nourished. The idea is entirely erroneous, and if practised is truly harmful, causing sour food deposits to accumulate in the intestines, and furthermore putting an additional burden on the blood-stream which is already overworked at such times, dealing with the excretions from the rapidly growing litter of puppies which, while in the womb, utilize the blood-stream of the dam in order to remove their own waste products. An in-whelp bitch requires extra milk for calcium provision; extra intake of water is also required to flush out the kidneys, which also bear part of the burden of ridding the body of the excretions of the developing litter. Clean water must always be available, day and night, removed only for an hour following meals.

Further attention should be paid to an abundant supply of natural mineral salts—supplied in the daily ration of raw green herbs, whole-grain cereals, and, to some extent, by the raw meat. For this purpose I have evolved a formula giving the most minerals rich in vegetation of land and sea. Nettles, comfrey and seaweed, all blended into a powder for giving on the raw meat. These tablets, fed daily to the bitch throughout the nine-weeks' in-whelp period, give amazing results, not only in general improvement of the litter, but in overcoming such in-whelp ailments as streptococcal infection, acid or failing milk, and so forth.

Special attention must be paid to the diet immediately before whelping. The litter has ceased growing by the beginning of the

Care of the In-whelp Bitch

eighth week, external furnishing such as nails and hair being mainly the only developing organs, and in general the puppies are very restless and active in preparation for the leaving of the womb. At such a time the organism of the dam does not want to be burdened with much food digestion; a gentle laxative diet should be aimed at for the last week of the in-whelp period. Meat supply should be reduced, and a main meal of raw milk, oats, or barley fed up to one or two days before the actual birth, when the bitch should be placed entirely on a fluid diet, a diet of milk and honey —average quantity is one teaspoon of honey to a large breakfast-cupful of milk. A toy-breed bitch would require on an average of one small cupful of milk and honey twice per day. A large breed about a half-pint or more per meal. Any reliable unadulterated make of that wonderful tree-bark flour food, slippery elm or red elm tree-flour food is a very helpful aid to bitches at such times, and has been utilized by hundreds of breeders, always with great success. Such food is also the ideal diet for the two days following whelping, when, as with immediately preceding whelping, no solid food should be given under any circumstances. This feeding of an entirely fluid diet immediately before and after whelping has done an immeasurable amount of good in reducing loss of life through whelping complications. The theory of such a measure is a sound one, it being that when the forces of the body are freed from the necessity of food digestion, they are at liberty for any other purpose of which the body may have need. For instance, during disease treatment, total fasting is employed in order to release the body powers for the processes of the cleansing of the blood-stream and the speedy removal of all disease toxins, and the subsequent repair of body tissues damaged in the interval of disease. In the case of the in-whelp bitch, all of the forces of the body can be concentrated on the birth of the puppies, and the prevention of the development of any fever conditions—which sometimes affect bitches which are not in total health, with the subsequent attack of puerperal fever and other allied ailments of birth.

The body has also much work to do, following the whelping, in the production of a good alkaline toxin-free milk flow and the shrinkage to natural size of the stretched organs of birth. There is also the complete expulsion of the products of after-birth to be dealt with.

Mention should be made here of that wonderful aid to easy

Care of the In-whelp Bitch

whelping, the wild raspberry-leaf plant. I was the first to popularize this herb among dog breeders, and the herb is now in habitual use as a whelping aid in kennels in all parts of the world. The popularity of the herb grew solely out of results obtained. When hitherto proved difficult whelpers whelped normal litters easily and speedily, following treatment with the herb, it was understandable that breeders should spread the news far and wide. In my veterinary-treatment files I have hundreds of reports from breeders supplying details of hitherto undreamt-of successful whelpings, especially from owners of the notoriously difficult whelping breeds, such as most of the toy breeds, the miniature breeds, and the big-headed bulldog-type breeds. The action of the herb on the organs of re-production is mainly tonic; hence its further use for sluggish stud dogs. The North American Indians, gypsies, and other races with a profound knowledge of herbal medicine, have long prescribed raspberry-leaf brew as an important medicine for pregnant women. A gypsy herbal document advises: 'Let all creatures with young, human and animal, take freely of raspberry herb. They will have very easy "times", and will be saved a tremendous amount of suffering.' Harold Ward, in his book, *Herbal Manual* (for humans), states: 'Thompson and his immediate successors strongly advised the free drinking of raspberry leaves infusion for several months before confinement as an aid to parturition, and it is still in much demand.'

This book has no space for publication in detail of breeders' reports—the book would grow to impossible length—but the use of raspberry leaf being of such importance to canine well-being, and the birthright of every brood bitch, I have made an exception here. Miss Florence Cockayne is an Irish terrier breeder, at Gorton, Suffolk (England), and is a hospital-trained nurse (St. Thomas's). 'As for raspberry leaves, I've never seen such easy whelpings until I used this herb, and the mothers keep so well during pregnancy, bowel evacuation being perfect. Bitches with their first litters give no trouble, the puppies being whelped effortlessly and with no pain. I sent some raspberry leaves on to a bulldog breeder in New South Wales, and she was absolutely amazed at the results; she had always had such ghastly times with her bitches, some of them sometimes being three days in labour. I had a Pekinese bitch who had had two miscarriages, but after having raspberry brew, carried her puppies full time and hardly knew that she was whelping.'

Care of the In-whelp Bitch

Mrs. S. Bancroft-Wilson, *Dog World*, England, pug correspondent and breeder of the Longlands pugs, also sends me a typical report: 'I have had wonderful results from the raspberry-leaf herb; breeding as I do from small well-boned bitches, I find the herb causes them to whelp quickly and easily. *I consider it is little short of miraculous.*'

Interest in raspberry herb has had a world-revival in recent years; so much so that the very conservative human medical journals have devoted articles to the use of this herb in childbirth, though such articles in the main—as is usually the case when reference to crude herbs is made in the chemical drug-dominated medical journals—were scornful, attesting any alleged merits to the mere psychological sphere of influence.

We who have studied the ways of the wild animals know that in the springtime they seek out various pregnancy plants, especially the early leaves and shoots of the wild raspberry and wild rose, chamomile, feverfew, and pennyroyal. Springtime is the natural breeding time for animals. The female carnivores, preying on the herb-eating animals, and, above all, seeking the herb-rich intestines of their prey, would quite surely get a sufficiency of pregnancy herbs to keep their own reproductive system in good clean health and aid the birth process of their offspring.

Before leaving the subject of raspberry-leaf herb, it should be mentioned how greatly the herb is associated with the reproductive organs, it being noticed at the time of whelping of bitches treated with raspberry that placentas are very dark green and, further, the presence of the strong and unmistakable odour of raspberry leaf is present throughout the time of the actual whelping and associated with the birth discharge. Many breeders have commented on this.

However, even raspberry leaf will not produce a normal and easy whelping if exercise is neglected. At least two hours' free (unleashed) exercise on clean land is essential throughout the in-whelp months, and also frequent daily walks.

RETENTION OF PUPPIES

It is general for the carnivores to give birth to their whelps easily and speedily. But sometimes an ill-placed puppy—or in an

57

Care of the In-whelp Bitch

unhealthy bitch, the whole litter—may be retained. Again, it is of great importance that the in-whelp bitch should be at the peak of good health, for in the case of abnormalities such as this there is then little risk of septic conditions developing. It is usually sufficient to give strong doses of raspberry-leaf herbs at four-hourly intervals for several days: two tablespoonfuls of powdered or finely minced raspberry herb, plus one dessertspoonful of molasses or black treacle, liquefied with sufficient warm water and given to the bitch (by forced drenching if necessary, for raspberry is a bitter-tasting herb when given in large doses). In cases of retained puppies, the bitch must be fasted until all are expelled. Semi-fasting is permissible, on a three-meal-per-day diet of milk and honey. In very severe cases of retained whelps, two tablespoonfuls of a brew of pennyroyal herb, plus one tablespoonful of Epsom salts dissolved in the brew of herb, should be given as a drench of one small cupful thrice daily. Drinks of linseed tea, given with the milk-honey meals, are helpful. If unsuccessful, surgery will be necessary.

RETENTION OF AFTERBIRTH

Retention of afterbirth is more common to the cow, goat, or ewe than to the dog, as bitches have to pass only small placentas, which leave their bodies easily. But in the case of retention in old bitches or in some species of the toy breeds, a brew made from one to three ivy leaves boiled up in a cupful of cold water, then allowed to brew for two hours, is a proved remedy. I always feed a handful of fresh ivy leaves to every goat as soon as she has given birth to her kid or kids. Dosage of ivy brew is two dessertspoons every three hours. If a bitch shows any discomfort following the birth of puppies, put her on a liquid diet of honey and water, or honey-milk-water, for several days.

DIET OF THE NURSING BITCH

This diet is identical with the in-whelp diet, except for increased rations, now that the bitch is free of the extra excretory burden hitherto imposed upon her by the litter developing within her womb. An additional early morning meal of fluid food, milk with honey and tree-barks flour, can be given if the litter is a large one. Oats should form the bulk of the cereal food as they are more

Care of the In-whelp Bitch

breast-milk-forming, and have more assimilable and concentrated protein than any other cereal for this purpose.

A healthy bitch should be able to feed her litter—large or small —for nine weeks. The Arabs reckon that a healthy lactation corresponds—at its minimum—to the duration of pregnancy. Thus the bitch will feed her litter for nine weeks or more, the human mother for at least nine months. But on modern unnatural diet a bitch's milk is often failing or acid at four weeks, and the human mother has to resort to devitalizing dried milk for her offspring.

TO INCREASE MILK RAPIDLY. All of the following foods are known to make milk. Unpasteurized cow or goat milk, grated raw carrot, cooked carrot (mashed), oat flakes, wholewheat, rye, bean-meal, seaweed powder (has been proved to increase butterfat content in milk in all animals, especially dairy cows), black treacle or molasses, honey, raw eggs, linseed tea, calamus root, pine kernels, dill seed, slippery-elm flour, marshmallow root (the three latter all obtainable in tree-barks-blend flour), finely cut borage leaves mixed in with the milk and sprinkled on the meat, and, lastly, an abundance of drinking-water.

The gun-dog expert Mrs. K. Wentworth-Smith (of the Yelme Golden Retrievers, Thelford, Norfolk, England) and her kennel manageress (Miss Eva B. Todd) have sent me a very comprehensive and interesting report on the effects of herbal medicine and natural rearing on the Yelme brood bitches: 'After many years of rigid adherence to natural feeding, combined with herbal additions, I am more than delighted with the result.

'In the case of in-whelp and nursing bitches the difference is most marked. The bitches retain their full health, spirits, and activity (as far as this latter is possible), produce their puppies with no distress, even if it is a first litter at five years old. Lactation is good, the bitches are willing, nay, anxious, to suckle their puppies so long as a drop of milk remains—the flow usually continuing abundant for at least *ten to twelve weeks*. Then, without exception, they follow Nature's design in vomiting up for their litter the food necessary to follow the milk diet. In fact, it is difficult to persuade them to renounce their maternal cares at all.

'During this period our experience is that the bitches retain their own well-being and vitality and are still well covered instead of having that "pulled-down" look, nor do they lose their dark pigmentation; in fact, this is even more marked.

Care of the In-whelp Bitch

'This method, by following the full cycle of Nature's design, also appears to ensure the brood bitch regaining her pre-birth neat and elegant figure—no unsightly or vulnerable "undercarriage" remaining to destroy symmetry, reduce activity, and get torn or injured when at field work.'

Medicines. A healthy bitch does not require medicines, especially not the general concoctions of the chemist. But Nature herself has provided a few plants which are of use in helping milk flow—marshmallow plant, flowers or leaves, is highly recommended for increasing the milk flow, so also is fennel herb, seeds or leaves, and borage, already described. Grated raw carrot given on the meat feed is also excellent. Also raw chopped dates given with the cereal feed. Raw eggs—but not more than three per week—are beneficial for this purpose. The milk flow can be used as an anti-worm aid for the suckling puppies if garlic is fed to the bitch daily throughout the nursing period. The penetrative powers of garlic are well known and well proved. The volatile oils of the garlic plant possess the unique powers of entering almost every cell of the body; but especially the body fluids, blood, urine, and, in the case of the female, the milk flow. It is well known what great care farmers take to keep their milking cows away from all contact with the garlic plant. I was intrigued to read in Thomas Hardy's great novel, *Tess of the D'Urbervilles*—which, incidentally, is a masterpiece of country-life description—how all the milkmaids are detailed off to search the meadows for a few single garlic plants which had entered and rooted in the meadow, and which were flavouring the milk yield of the entire herd of a hundred or more cattle—so powerful is the garlic plant's power of milk-flow penetration, and so equally powerful the kine's natural desire to partake of the wonderfully medicinal herb whenever the plant grows within reach. Garlic dosage will serve the additional purpose of keeping the bitch herself worm-free during the vital time of the nursing and, later, the weaning of her puppies.

DISTEMPER (see Chapter 6). An in-whelp bitch that develops distemper, treated by internal-cleansing method, can whelp a perfectly normal litter. I have nursed many in-whelp bitches through distemper, for breeders, and have seen excellent litters with no sign at all of their mother's disease.

FEVER. Fever of the puerperal type is not common in bitches. But if a case should occur, then immediate strong dosing with

Care of the In-whelp Bitch

herbal antiseptic tablets is required, and fasting on honey-water. Give a nightly laxative, of senna pods preferably. The litter must be removed from the dam, and hand-fed. The dam's milk must be expressed by hand three times daily. When the fever subsides and the bitch is back on a solid-foods diet, her puppies can be restored.

ECLAMPSIA. The bitch may sometimes suffer from a glandular disturbance generally known as eclampsia. The theory much in vogue with dog breeders is that this disorder (a form of epileptic fits or severe total body cramp) is caused solely by calcium deficiency in the blood. The mineral which is actually lacking in most cases is iodine; the only healthful way of supplying this in its natural organic form is in the cells of most seaweeds and some vegetables. The giving of chemical iodine is unnatural and very harmful. In the rarer cases, when it is indeed calcium drainage, injection of calcium into the blood-stream is the quickest cure. Neglected eclampsia can cause death.

MASTITIS. This condition is not very common in the canine race for, unlike the domestic cow or goat, the bitch is allowed to suckle her offspring as Nature intended, and is not subjected to milking machines, and so forth. The ailment is most commonly caused by feeble puppies who are unable to suckle their dam strongly and therefore do not empty the breasts several times daily. Congestion results and mastitis develops. The typical symptom is swelling and hardness of the whole milk-secreting area, and often a few degrees of fever. The bitch usually refuses to allow the puppies to feed from her because of the pain caused by the congestion.

Treatment. The puppies should be removed from the bitch and, meantime, hand-reared. The milk glands must be emptied of all milk by hand expression, first applying cloths dipped in hot water to the breasts. This should be carried out four to five times during the day. The milk-glands area should be bathed with a brew of elder and dock leaves—one handful of each brewed in 1½ pints of water. Internal treatment is one day's complete fast on water only, with four herbal antiseptic tablets given twice daily (average breed); a laxative in the evening, then a fluid diet of milk and honey for several days until normality is restored. The puppies can then feed again from their dam. This treatment, which I originated for cows and goats, gave very good results for these animals and was much recommended by that great farmer, Sir Albert Howard.

Care of the In-whelp Bitch

GENERAL TREATMENT OF THE BROOD BITCH

A brood bitch requires careful treatment, both psychological and practical. General treatment not only affects the bitch's own health but, further, has an important bearing upon the health of the litter, both before and after birth. I will deal first with the psychological handling.

I absolutely deplore the turning of any animal into a mere breeding machine, but especially so the dog, because of its great capacity for affection towards its human master, and its great gifts of intelligence, both practical and spiritual. Throughout England there are dozens of kennels that keep their bitches virtually prisoners: year after year they are brought out of prison confinement for mating and whelping, and then sent back again to the long months of mental boredom, their world of no larger interest than that of a wooden kennel and a concrete run (for persons who keep their dogs as kennel prisoners usually favour the concrete run: it is simpler to keep 'clean' than the more healthful brick or natural grass run). It is no wonder, following such treatment, that the offspring of pedigree stock has acquired the popular reputation of being 'idiots'. In my eyes the brood bitch should be looked upon as a highly important, and therefore privileged, person. This is only rightful when it is appreciated that the future continuance of any particular strain of dog is greatly dependent upon the health and the breeding powers of the brood bitch.

Throughout the in-whelp period the bitch requires increased human companionship and an extra amount of exercise, so that she is kept mentally alert and active. A feeling of absolute trust must be developed between owner and bitch, so that in the case of any whelping complications arising the bitch will yield her body with an absolutely calm mind to the care of the human owner (this factor is of tremendous importance in the saving of a bitch and her litter in freak or complicated whelpings). Also such relationship removes all risks of a bitch savaging her puppies, which event in almost every case—and it is common enough in general dog breeding—is purely a matter of nervous hysteria. The bitch should be given all protection from alarming noises when with her litter, and she should never be compelled to soil her bed. I have known kennel owners with nursing bitches leave their kennels for

Care of the In-whelp Bitch

a full day while attending dog shows, leaving bitches confined with their litters in closed kennels. Such absolute cruelty appears to be quite habitual in general dog breeding. Is it then to be wondered at that many bitches savage their puppies?

Practical treatment is dependent on correct diet, as already described, and frequent, regular, and abundant daily exercise. For the first few days, of course, very little exercise is required, but the bitch must be allowed away from her litter at frequent intervals in order to stretch her limbs, pass urine, and cleanse her bowels. Also at such times her lungs are panting for abundant draughts of fresh out-of-doors' air. Regular daily grooming is also an essential, both to keep her body clean and to assist complete circulation of the blood; thorough daily grooming is also very beneficial to the nervous system. To assist general body cleansing, the fasting treatment is also to be utilized. A regular weekly half-day fast, instead of the usual weekly whole-day adult fast, is sufficient, with one whole day per month. The one whole day per month, both during the in-whelp period and the nursing period, is *essential* to true total health and must not be neglected.

It is natural for the in-whelp bitch to fast on the day she is due to whelp and for at least twenty-four hours following whelping. Cats will often refuse all food for two or three days after they have given birth to their kittens.

Domestication has changed this and altered natural instincts. The body has no time or forces to expend on food digestion during the important time of birth, nor immediately following birth when the temporarily weakened system requires strengthening, not through unwanted heavy foods, but through rest, sleep, and absolute quiet.

At the most, brood bitches can be fed milk and honey on the day due to whelp, and very watered milk and honey during the day following whelping. Then introduce cereal feeds and milk. Do not give a heavy meal of meat until the third day after whelping. In cases of exhaustion, fresh grape juice (or, if not available, then bottled grape juice) can be given as a medicine every two hours or so. An average amount would be two tablespoons for a medium-size bitch. Give also honey.

When whelping is prolonged in the case of big litters, one puppy only should be left with the mother while she is whelping; the others, after cleaning by the dam, should be placed apart on a warm bottle covered by a blanket from contact with the puppies, to await the arrival of all the litter.

Leaving puppies under the mother when whelping may cause fatalities. In the wild the death of several puppies is probably accounted for by Nature; in professional breeding the best of the litter may be lost accidentally this way.

3

Care of Puppies in the Nest

Very little attention to suckling puppies is required, from the time of birth until the commencement of weaning in the third to fourth week. If the bitch is in normal health, she will keep the puppies clean, warm, and well nourished without any human interference. Indeed, the more the bitch is left in quiet solitude, the better it is for the litter. It is the bitch alone who requires attention, and such care has been described in the preceding chapter.

The docking of tails and the removal of dew-claws in the chosen breeds should be carried out as early as possible—around the third day in healthy puppies. The wounds must not be dressed with iodine or any chemical disinfectant, most of which retard healing and are the frequent cause of puppy losses at such times. Use preferably witch-hazel extract—which is purely herbal—or a herbal brew made from elder-tree leaves, or blackberry leaves, or whole sprigs of rosemary or rue. (To make the herbal brew: finely shred two tablespoons of freshly gathered, preferably, or dry leaves or flowering sprigs of the above-mentioned herbs, scald with $\frac{1}{2}$ pint of boiling water, allow to brew overnight, then strain and use cold. Thoroughly bathe the wounded areas with the herbal brew.)

Puppies in the nest should be kept in the semi-dark until their eyes have opened. The building housing them must be absolutely clean and well ventilated. Dirty kennels are the cause of the loss of far more newly born puppies than ever die from disease. Breeders habitually keep litters in much-used kennels, where the wooden boards are urine-soaked and worm- and various bacteria-impregnated. Kennels used for puppy-rearing purposes *must* be regularly long-term rested and whitewashed. To put successive litters into the same kennels is simply inviting general disease development. A clean, rested, newly whitewashed kennel must be

65

used for each litter reared. Blankets as bedding should be avoided; newspaper is far better.

HAND REARING. This is an unnatural process and really should have no place in this book on natural rearing. Every bitch should be able to rear her own litter without human interference. However, breeders at various times have had to hand-rear an odd litter, and natural-rearing principles of diet have been applied with great success. Indeed, bench champions have been produced from such rearings.

It is impossible to give rules for feeding times. The new-born puppies being suckled by their dam feed whenever hungry and sleep away the rest of the time. But feeds should be very frequent for the first week: two-hourly by day and four-hourly by night. Diet should be essentially natural foods, raw cow or goat milk diluted with water from flaked oats which have been soaked overnight, and honey. To every cup of milk add two dessertspoons oats water, one small teaspoon of honey and a few drops of almond, corn or sesame oil. This mixture should be given tepid— do not spoil the milk by overheating it. Chamomile herb tea is very soothing and can be used for soaking the oat flakes. Use a small feeding-bottle with a finely pierced rubber teat. In the second week, a little N.R. tree-barks gruel can be added to the milk for extra soothing power and for increased vitamins and minerals. Numerous animals of many kinds have been hand-reared on this food. Not only puppies and kittens, but also goat kids, lambs, young owls and hawks—all achieved great health on bottle-fed feeds of goat's milk and tree-barks slippery-elm flour. A mere pinch of this flour per puppy, at first, increasing to a half and then a whole teaspoon as the puppies grow on. They should also be fed drinks of barley water, several times daily, for its slightly laxative and further soothing properties. This should be made by pouring hot (not boiled) water over whole grain barley, allowing this to stand overnight, and then expressing the liquid through a piece of muslin.

The puppies must be kept warm with the aid of a well-blanketed hot-water bottle. Their anal and bladder areas should be kept clean with cotton wool swabs dipped into warm water, squeezed semi-dry, and then a little olive oil applied; a good talcum powder is also useful. Clean the puppies after every feed.

A loud-ticking alarm-clock, wrapped in a cloth, gives orphaned animals the impression that their mother is with them.

Care of Puppies in the Nest

Puppies hand-reared this way seldom scour, do not develop potbellies, and are very active and contented.

AILMENTS OF THE NEW-BORN LITTER

Puppies in the nest generally remain immune from the major ailments such as distemper, nervous diseases, and other ailments of the adult dog. The principal disorders of early puppyhood are: 'fading' disease, now usually attributed to beta haemolytic streptococcal disease (b.h.s.), although sometimes this may be brought on by a toxic or very acid milk flow of the dam; dysentery, or scouring, worm infestation—especially by wireworms, which can frequently kill off very young puppies—skin disorders, especially mange. For detailed curative treatments, readers are referred to Part Two of this book where the ailments are separately and fully dealt with, both preventative and curative treatments being given. In Part Two there is an especially large section on streptococcal disease. For cure of this now very common canine ailment, my internal cleansing herbal treatment has been immensely successful, having overcome the disease in many of Europe's famous kennels.

COCCIDIOSIS. Sera and chemical drug treatments completely failed to cure streptococcal disease. There has had to be found some scapegoat for the failure of the expensive orthodox treatments inflicted on the harassed dog breeders. When unnatural treatments have failed to cure the streptococcal infection—indeed, in many cases have aggravated the trouble—some reason must be forthcoming for the failure; and now, therefore, breeders are being told that there is yet a new canine ailment responsible for barren bitches or fading out of litters: this is *Coccidiosis*! Cocci are single spherical-shaped bacteria (in contrast to the streptococci bacteria which are found in chains); just as with streptococci, they are very common, and are very widely distributed; they can, likewise, be found in perfectly healthy body tissue. Coccidiosis has long been a bugbear in goat, rabbit, and poultry breeding, but hitherto it has not been given much publicity in canine medicine, streptococcal disease dominating the stage. I advise all intelligent dog breeders to treat this ailment in the exact way that they are treating b.h.s. Remove the root cause of the disease by replacing unnatural rearing methods by natural ones, and by treating the actual ailment entirely on the system advocated for streptococcal disease, which treatment has been so unfailingly successful. Professor M. Perek, D.V.M., of the Agricultural Faculty of the Hebrew University, Jerusalem, told me that one of his workers demonstrated that coccidiosis in poultry could be cured with the use of garlic given to the infected birds.

DYSENTERY (DIARRHOEA, SCOURING). Sometimes very young puppies, perhaps under one week of age, begin scouring—usually a grey or pale yellow diarrhoea. Unless this trouble is checked the puppies will die. General treatment is: remove the litter from the dam for two days, give six small meals per day (hand-rearing) of very diluted tepid water and honey: about one-quarter teaspoonful of honey to one dessertspoonful tepid (unboiled) water, at each meal, average-size breeds. Give one leaf-extract tablet, crushed into small pieces, average-size breed. Bigger dose for older puppies. Or give a tea of bilberry leaves. Then after two days, return litter to the dam, who herself should have been fasted for at least one day and dosed with leaf-extract tablets—treatment of the dam being followed as a precautionary measure in case it is her milk which is causing the litter to scour. Needless to say, the litter must be kept very warm throughout the time of the removal from the dam, using flannel-covered hot-water bottles; and they must be kept clean with olive oil applied on cotton wool, with talcum powder used in order to prevent skin chafing and soreness. If the scouring returns, then the treatment must be repeated at short intervals. This treatment has saved hundreds of very sick litters, and puppies so treated have grown into healthy adults.

The litter should be weaned strictly on tree-barks food flour, which has stomachic and intestinal healing properties.

'FADING OUT' of young puppies. This trouble is fully dealt with under the Streptococcal Disease section in Part Two. At the present time, hepatitis is largely blamed for puppy losses. General treatment is through the dam, pre-natal and post-natal. The following report is of interest, from Mrs. Winifred Barber, journalist and judge, writing in *Our Dogs*, Scottish Terrier breed notes. 'Miss Gwen Southwell reports: "I read your notes a few weeks ago about bitches missing, etc., and there has been a lot of talk about puppies fading out, so I thought I would tell you of my experience with my winning Fox Terrier bitch, Fulgents Nigella. I have for some time been interested in herbal remedies, and about six weeks before she had her litter I gave her one leaf-extract tablet a day. She had four dogs and one bitch, all sturdy, lovely puppies, yet they seemed a bit discontented, although they fed well. On the fourth day one of the dogs became distended and very uncomfortable. . . ." [A typical condition of 'fading out'.—J. de B.-L.] "I thought that he was going to become a 'wailer' and that I should lose him—it used to be quite a common thing for me to lose one in this way before the war. However, I gave the mother four leaf-extract tablets (they are wonderful for any sign of strep.), and two garlic herbal tablets a day, and next day the puppy was normal and all have gone on very well since . . . the dam continued to have a herbal tablet every day. Since weaning, the puppies have had a ten-day course, and I haven't seen a sign of a worm from them. My puppies always had lots in the old days. I am so pleased to have saved my puppy. I hope that my experience may be of use to others; it is so disappointing when they fade out." '

PUPPY SKIN RASH. This skin rash is not to be confused with follicular mange, with which skin ailment many puppies are born, coming into life already infected from the dam; this follicular condition is quite often found in smooth-haired dachshunds, litters being born totally devoid of hair. In such cases the skin has a blue-grey hue and is sweaty to the feel and is also evil-smelling. This is totally different from the rash which sometimes affects unweaned puppies, bred from a bitch that is not in normal health. The skin ailment is often called 'milk-rash' and is typified by crusty scabs covering large areas, sometimes the entire body. The body hair is not generally lost. Treatment is internal with leaf extract, average one crushed tablet per puppy per day, plus external bathing of the body surface with cotton-wool swabs dipped into a brew of blackberry leaves. The blackberry lotion is wonderfully effective in treatment of all eczematous conditions. Clover flowers, and/or leaves, or elder blossom can be added to the brew with much benefit.

WORM INFESTATION. Worm infestation in newly born puppies is a very fatal condition and often results in early death, especially if the worms are of the wire variety. This trouble would never happen if the dam received proper pre-natal treatment and was in sound health at the time of whelping. But it is freely acknowledged that the ova of worms can circulate in the blood-stream of the dam and thus reach the bodies of the unborn puppies, so that the litter is infested before birth. Treatment must be carried out, firstly,

Care of Puppies in the Nest

through the dam, who should be dosed with herbal worm tablets. In severe infestation of puppies, give them one tablet (average dose) cut up small, then follow the worm tablets, fifteen minutes later, with a dessertspoon dose of Milk of Magnesia, which has use as a mild laxative, but I do not advise as an antacid in canine use. Or senna laxative can be given: one large pod soaked in one dessertspoon of cold water for approximately four hours; a pinch of powdered ginger should be added to this. This is for one puppy.

I must here stress that there is no advantage at all in blasting out by means of various chemicals (bowel irritants mostly) vast numbers of worms; the injury thus caused is twice that which the worms themselves are able to cause, worms in general feeding on the mucus and other impurities accumulated in the intestines. The aims should be to remove those impurities on which the worms are feeding and in which they have imbedded themselves. Remove the impurities first by the aid of that proved internal cleanser, herbal garlic, rue, etc., via the mother's milk, and then by a laxative and restorative weaning diet—especially a dict of whole raw foods.

WEANING

It is impossible to give strict rules for puppy weaning, as weaning differs greatly with individual breeds, and even with individual puppies. But I can say with authority that hurried weaning, careless weaning, unnatural weaning can ruin a puppy's health, so that ever afterwards there is a predisposition to fits, hysteria, gastritis, worm infestation. It is worth taking all possible care. It is a matter of true personal breeding skill to know what exact quantities of food to feed to individual puppies, also when to feed and when to fast—for fasting should play an important part in all animal rearing, although that measure is usually totally ignored by the majority of breeders.

On one subject, however, it is possible to speak very precisely, and that is concerning the correct time for weaning. One of the greatest errors of Western dog weaning (and also child weaning) is the general haste to get the puppies to partake of solid food. In dog breeding the great incentive appears to be commercial, i.e. the earlier the weaning, likewise the earlier the puppies can be offered for sale. Slow weaning as opposed to hasty weaning is a necessity, because Nature has not prepared the intestines and

Care of Puppies in the Nest

stomachs of infant carnivores for the digestion of anything other than milk food until or after the fourth week. Food—especially the usual starchy white-flour puppy-weaning foods fed to the puppy before the fourth week—will be digested to some extent, but at the same time it is distending the stomach and intestines and creating acid condition of the blood-stream and a sour mucus-laden condition of the digestive organs; thus making an ideal state for the development of worm ova, streptococcal bacteria, and distemper disease. Wean the puppies in their fourth week on raw goat or cow milk thickened with honey. Milk should be fed tepid to cold, never hot. Then for extra feeding value, strengthen the milk with a preparation of slippery-elm tree-barks flour, making sure that the slippery elm is pure and unrefined. Slippery elm is not a cheap substance, and consequently some manufacturers of this food, wanting to make the high profits common to commercial foods, add such quantities of cheap white flour to the elm that the food becomes nothing more than flour flecked with particles of elm bark. The genuine preparation, as I sell it, is a brown colour with a very strong, characteristic smell.

I once met a well-known North England breeder of wire fox terriers, who was a long-time sufferer from gastric disease, and on his doctor's advice was on a diet of milk and slippery-elm food. He had made no progress in curing his ailment. I asked him to send me a sample of the elm food which he was taking. I soon saw that the food was a useless commercial product, flour adulterated beyond chance of possessing any curative properties. I therefore sent a supply of the genuine, natural product, and the improvement in the man's health was instant and remarkable, gastric pain disappeared and he began to feel marvellously well. I am relating this now to point out the importance of ascertaining that foods used are in a natural state as opposed to the general over-refined or adulterated products wherein the natural properties of the ingredients are almost totally removed during manufacture. (The reasons for interference with natural foods are manifold. To enhance the keeping properties of food is a very usual reason—in short, to enable the selling of stale products; or to lower the manufacturers' own production costs and to increase their trade profits. For instance, in the processing of natural wheat grain, big side profits are to be made from the sale of the bran and of the wheat germ—the extraction of the vital 'life' of the wheat in its

Care of Puppies in the Nest

germ also enhances the long-term keeping properties of the resultant flours, important for profitable commerce.)

Mention should here and now be made of that other commonly spoiled, vitally important, puppy-weaning food—milk. For milk to be true food, it should be raw, unheated fluid food from healthy goats or cows. The sterilizing of milk in pasteurization, and likewise the drying of milk to turn it into powder form, both destroy the vital vitamin and cosmic properties which are so peculiar to milk and are so very delicate therein. The milk of herbivorous animals is—or should be—mainly the vitamin-rich herbage and vegetable matter on which the animal has been feeding, in general liquid suspension. (Note how quickly and surely such high-tasting foods as garlic, various root vegetables, and other plants—the milk of clover-fed cattle is honey-sweet to the taste—enters the milk flow.) All leaf matter contains vital forces other than vitamins. Professor Dr. Szekely describes these forces as 'cosmic'; they come to the plant from the radiations from sun, moon, and stars; the forces contain great restorative, regenerative, and healing powers; in raw, natural, untreated milk most of these forces—so vital to health—are found intact. There is no substitute for clean, raw milk. I appreciate that such food is difficult to obtain at present, but if people want to breed dogs they should make adequate preparations for the proper feeding of same; they should keep goats. For instance, who but an idiot would attempt to rear a horse without having any grazing ground available for the animal? And yet hundreds of breeders mate their bitches and proceed to rear a litter without having made any provision for the supplying of those foodstuffs vital to true and normal health. No wonder that puppy losses are so prevalent nowadays, and subhealth is the general rule among most pedigreed dogs rather than the exception.

The following two opinions on milk as a food will uphold my own findings on the subject. Firstly, from Dr. John Harvey Kellogg's treatise, *Auto-Intoxication*: 'Milk is a sort of fluid tissue and like other tissues is prepared from the blood; hence it is not surprising that the profound scientific study to which this remarkable food substance has been subjected within recent years has brought to light the fact that milk possesses some of the properties of the living blood from which it is produced. While still warm with animal heat *freshly drawn milk, like the blood, possesses the power to combat and destroy germs.* Milk contains various anti-

Care of Puppies in the Nest

bodies which are found in the blood, agglutins, anti-toxins, and opsonins. It must be admitted that these last-named elements of milk have been so recently discovered that their relation and value to human life and health are not yet fully understood.'

From the *Daily Telegraph*: 'Dr. Sanderson-Wells, of the Food Education Society, described at a meeting in London yesterday, an experiment by a research worker, who devised a perfectly balanced chemical meal containing all the necessary vitamins on which he fed a number of rats. All the rats died. Another professor added one tablespoon of fresh milk to the chemical meal and the rats to which he fed it all thrived. When the milk was boiled before adding it to the meal, all the rats died. Ill-feeding, said the doctor, was the basis of all disease.'

As the puppies approach their fifth week the milk food should be thickened with whole-grain flaked cereals, making a beginning with flaked barley which is the most simple cereal from a digestive point of view. If not obtainable, use flaked oats. Soon the first teeth will be felt in the gums.

Now at this time, towards the fifth week, raw meat should be introduced. The natural instinct of the bitch when in the wild state (and common to all carnivores) is to semi-digest flesh food in her own stomach, and then to vomit up the food for the use of her whelps. Therefore, keeping this in mind, it should be understood that some preparation of the meat will be necessary. Early preparation of meat is simply the rendering of it in as easily digestible form as possible, by means *other than* cooking. The meat should be hung for some time before use in order to soften it, and only lean meat should be fed at first. A big slice should be selected and the surface then scraped with a knife, the soft red flesh which then adheres to the blade of the knife or the edge of the spoon (a spoon can be used for meat scraping) should then be removed and fed to the puppy in bulk. Ration for a first meal for an average-size puppy would be approximately one teaspoon. This quantity should be increased every three days, until, at eight weeks of age, the puppy (average-size breed) is having two tablespoons of finely shredded meat twice per day. By that time—eight weeks—the puppy will be fully weaned. The future diet of the growing puppy up to adult age has already been given in the Diet Charts at the end of Chapter 1.

Remember that every ounce, every particle of food contributes

73

Care of Puppies in the Nest

to the strength of puppy legs, therefore let every meal given be of maximum health in natural concentration and preparation.

A properly weaned puppy is a joy to see and possess. It has come into the world with a set of 'brand-new' organs: heart, brain, liver, kidneys, etc. All are new, clean, unspoiled. It is each puppy's right that it be fed foods which will not damage or degenerate its new body, but improve and safeguard its health, so that it will never know the pain and distress of worm infestation, rickets, scouring, skin eruptions. The great naturalist, W. H. Hudson, said of that natural-living race, the gypsies (before in-roads of civilization and faulty modern diet caused the health degeneration which has become prevalent among them today): 'I've never seen a gypsy with a cold, a headache, indigestion or backache. Wind, snow, rain, they maintain their splendid health.' I can say the same of a truly naturally reared puppy: I've never seen a sickly one or a weakly one; they flourish from the day of birth and are weaned as stalwart, independent little individuals, ready to play their important parts in the canine world.

Cleanliness is a first essential. The puppies should be cleanly housed, and bedded on good-quality hay or straw (preferably hay). For although hay bedding is supposed to encourage vermin, there are health-giving properties in the dry produce of green meadows not possessed by any other form of bedding; and in any case the firm skins and 'tough' body hair of really healthy puppies do not encourage insect parasites to linger there. Such vermin go farther afield for the weak-tissued, unhealthy skins of animals degenerate in health, for under such circumstances they can take a firm foothold from which they will not easily be dislodged until the death of the animal host. The persistence with which fleas and lice return again and again to the bodies of unhealthy animals, as soon as chemical warfare upon the skin vermin is relaxed by the breeder, has always impressed me. The growing puppies must have daily access to grassland. The dew which forms on clean, healthy grass—barren, sour grass lacks dew formation—is an important tonic for young puppies, and most puppies which have not totally lost their natural instincts will be found licking eagerly at the surface of dew or rain-wet herbage. The puppies' search for moisture indicates that a feed of water must be made available as soon as their eyes open. Water should always be present in the kennel run (not in the kennel, except with in-whelp bitches, which

74

Care of Puppies in the Nest

frequently require to partake of water during the night), other than shortly before or after meals. The partaking of water while food digestion is in progress both washes the food over quickly from the stomach down into the intestines and dilutes the digestive juices.

Sleep is as important to growing puppies as is good natural food. Young puppies should be put to sleep in well-ventilated kennels for several hours at a fixed hour during every day. They should also be put to bed early and given the great benefit of early rising. No breeder who is himself a late riser, and who habitually deprives his dogs of the benefits of the sweet vital air of the early-morning hours, will ever make a true success of dog rearing. As a university student, I acquired the bad habit of late-night study and consequent late-morning rising; it was dog ownership and the necessity of giving them the essential morning exercise which caused me to return to natural hours in keeping with the true laws of Nature. I love the early mornings, and nothing will ever again deprive me of them.

Puppies do not require sunlight on their bodies before their eyes are opened at their tenth to fourteenth day, and even afterwards they should be shaded from very strong sunlight until their newly opened eyes have strengthened. Very young puppies will scream lustily if exposed to very strong sunlight without any access to shade. When it is remembered that in the wild state they were sheltered in dark caves during the first weeks of their lives, the dislike of the young puppy for sunlight can be understood. But as soon as the puppies have reached the weaning stage, and their limbs have become active, then sunlight is one of the most important attributes to successful rearing. Indeed, it is an essential: as with a growing plant, no creature, apart from the nocturnal ones, can flourish when kept in the dark; sun is the supreme life-giver, for without sun there can be no life.

Puppies, from their early weeks, should be given separate dishes when weaned. Be strict concerning this, as competitive feeding causes overeating and thus digestive ailments. It is natural in the wild for each fox or wolf cub to run off with its portion of torn flesh and devour this at safe distance from the other cubs. Only by separate feeding can the owner be sure that each puppy receives its proper share of food.

75

4

General Notes on Natural Rearing

Throughout the preceding chapters of this book I have stressed the importance of diet in puppy rearing, for without proper diet you cannot rear healthy puppies. It is nonsense, for example, to advise adequate exercise if the puppy's limbs have been rendered too rachitic (rickety) from faulty diet to allow any exercise to be taken.

But in this chapter, assuming that proper diet is being followed, I am giving some well-proved hints on puppy care which will add to the well-being of all puppies. I have followed the plan of a book on horse breeding which I once used to study: this book was divided into two sections, 'The External Horse' and 'The Internal Horse'.

The external dealt with grooming, stable management, exercise, and so forth; the internal, with diet, disease prevention and cure, and so forth. I shall in this chapter follow something of that horse-book plan.

EXTERNAL CARE

GROOMING. Daily grooming is an essential of puppy rearing when stock is kennel raised. Yet I have known famous kennels (famous on show wins only) who never groom their stock except for show preparation. Grooming encourages hair growth, allows the hair—which, after all, is a living tissue—to breathe, keeps vermin in check, aids the circulation, and conditions the delicate nerve fibres which mass in the skin layers. Country-living dogs require less grooming than town ones, for in their daily exercise the herbage and bushes friction their bodies, and clean rain bathes

General Notes on Natural Rearing

them. Only in summertime they must be searched for skin vermin, especially grass ticks. I advocate for all dogs a weekly sponge-down with pine fluid (genuine, not synthetic), a few drops to a half pint of tepid water, and a monthly bath in soapy water, rinsing off very well. Use soap flakes, not detergents, and a bar of olive oil soap, such as Palmolive. More frequent bathing is essential for town dogs, grimed by chimney smoke and motor-vehicle fumes. No dog can enjoy true health when its body is coated with a film of grime.

An Afghan hound I had with me for three months in New York recently, required a weekly bath; and each week tubs of black water were washed from her golden coat.

Needless to say, all grooming equipment must also be washed at least weekly. It is useless to groom an animal with soiled combs and brushes. Bristle brushes and bone combs are far better for hair health than plastic ones. Collars and leads should also be cleaned regularly, using an oily rag or paraffin rag, and then polishing with leather polish.

Dogs must be examined regularly for presence of lice, fleas, ticks, or mange infections. Coats should be dusted frequently with a safe herbal insecticide. Never use poisons nor DDT preparations. They not only harm the eye and inner ears of dogs, but also settle on herbage and contaminate food, and act as insidious, if slow, poisons internally. Even such large mammals as rabbits have died from the use of DDT despite the commercial assurances that such chemicals are harmless to health. For fuller instructions for safe destruction of skin vermin, please see 'Fleas, Lice, Ticks, etc.', in Chapter 6.

Clean rain-water is a wonderful hair tonic, as also is dew. Exercise dogs in the rain frequently: a healthy dog loves rain. Dry down wet dogs with a dry wash-leather, which will absorb much moisture; newspaper can then be used to finish off, or handfuls of pine saw-dust on smooth-coated dogs. Then bed the dog on thick layers of newspaper which will dry him off completely. Wet cats should also be bedded on newspaper for drying them. A dog loves to cleanse itself as nature intended, by rolling its body on grass, but this cannot be achieved if the grass is that of a stale kennel run, urine soaked and dirty. My Afghan hounds, retaining their natural instincts from their mountain-living ancestors, take self-taught grooming sessions by rolling among thickets of fern or on

77

clumps of reeds. They do this deliberately, generation after generation.

An old-fashioned but excellent shampoo, for human as well as canine use, is raw eggs, although it proves expensive for other than toy breeds. M.B.F. Products, Wilton, Connecticut, U.S.A., makes a good, natural shampoo, containing eggs and yeast. It is reasonably priced and gives the coat a wonderful shine. It is much used for show dogs.

For a home-made shampoo, use four eggs to a pint of warm water, beating up the eggs very well in the water until the shampoo foams. To improve this yet further, a standard brew of rosemary plant is added to the eggs in place of plain water (see Chapter 5, Preparation of Herbs, pp. 94–96). Bathe dog first with an olive-oil soap, rinse off, and then, instead of the second soaping, use the egg shampoo. Rinse shampoo off the coat very well or it will adhere and spoil the fine shine which follows its proper use.

For grooming 'shine' on coats, an excellent daily finish-off to grooming is friction and polishing with a wash-leather dipped into cold common tea or a strong brew of rosemary herb. Or the bare hands can be dipped into tea or herbal brew and used to polish the coat; that is how the Arabs polish their Arabian horses and salukis, using often a weak brew of henna leaves. Nettle tea is also a famous old-fashioned coat tonic, used as a friction, making the hair shine and removing scurf. (Some nettle tea can also be given with benefit for internal use, by spoon or soaked into the cereal feed. Bring nettles to the boil in hot water, then remove from the boil and steep for two to three hours. Gloves must be used when cutting off the nettles, for they sting the skin at a touch before being boiled.)

SUNLIGHT. As I have said elsewhere in this book, without sun there can be no life. The maximum of sun for all animals should be a kennel rule, with also ample shade provided, so that the dog can himself choose his own natural sunbathing hours or seek shade, as he desires. Sunlight is not merely a tonic and restorative and a potent destroyer of bacteria, it is also a vital food. It is one of the main sources of vitamin A. It is understood that when a dog is seen to lick at its body hair after sunning itself, it is partaking of vitamin A, which collects on the hair surfaces; the dog is also seeking vital cosmic dust which comes earthwards on the sun's rays. *Sunlight is essential to natural puppy rearing*; there is no

General Notes on Natural Rearing

substitute for it, not electric sunlamps or anything else. Puppies reared indoors in apartments or sometimes even below ground level in basements, as is often done in big cities in America and elsewhere, can never possess true health, and their disease resistance is very low.

KENNELS. For nature rearing, kennels must be roomy, well ventilated, sunny, and dry. Artificial heating should be avoided; dogs, being of the wolf family, thrive in cold, but dislike damp. In very wet weather, the best dry warmth that man can provide for the domestic dog is a deep bed of dry litter, straw, hay, bracken, etc., in a draught-proof corner of the kennel. Pinewood sawdust or shavings on the floor give warmth and absorb damp.

Winter litters are unnatural. The female fox and wolf will not get themselves mated in the mid-year; they await the natural breeding time which ensures springtime whelping, to rear their whelps in the warmth of spring sunlight. If some heat is needed for young puppies which have been winter whelped, then a common paraffin-burning storm lantern, hung on a strong, long nail, to keep the lamp out of near contact with the wall, can be kept burning night and day. A storm lamp will give ample heat for any average-size kennel. Keep the lamp spotlessly clean, allowing no drop of paraffin to remain on it after filling, to cause fume smells. In the coldest mountain winters of Spain I have never needed other heating for my animals.

KENNEL RUNS. Daily contact, for long periods, with clean earth and grassland is another essential of N.R. puppy rearing. I have known puppies fed strictly on raw-foods diet and conditioned only with herbal medicines that still do not thrive, solely because they were being kept in stale kennel runs soiled by countless earlier litters. Puppies need a fresh or well-rested area of ground for each litter bred. Portable wire runs on wooden posts should be used, with the wire moved to a different piece of land every month, while the puppies are young and constantly soiling the runs. Unlike that of cattle, sheep and goats, the urine of dogs is bad for the soil. Stale earth runs should be dug over and well limed and then sown with fresh grass seed. I have known grass seed to refuse to grow at all in much-used dog runs, even after liming, so foul and sour had the earth been allowed to become. No wonder, therefore, that puppies which have been reared in such runs grow up to be sickly creatures, undersized and nervous.

General Notes on Natural Rearing

Miss A. N. Hartley, Rotherwood Deerhounds, who has reared so many stalwart champion hounds in this country, sums up the matter very well in a letter to me: 'Cleanliness, fresh air and exercise, and good food, have always been my four essentials of puppy rearing. I agree with you most heartily in believing that having too many dogs on a small area spells inevitable disaster. The dogs and runs are consequently not then kept really clean, with the result that bacteria find good living quarters.

'Far too many people believe that dog breeding is a pleasant hobby with which to make money in one's spare time, and this spells overcrowding and neglect of the dogs.'

Vernon Hirst, famed terrier man and judge, of England, gives sound advice: 'I am a believer in letting my bitches and puppies run on natural ground, and did not have my runs concreted. I used to place a nice-sized board inside the run for them to lie on when at rest in good weather. I tried to keep as near to the natural as possible, and the result was I escaped many illnesses.'

EXERCISE. Early morning and evening exercise is best. Do not exercise in the full heat of a summer day or immediately after meals. For true health, allow all dogs to enjoy exercise in all weathers, wind, rain, snow. Leash exercise is almost valueless. A dog needs to run and leap, and thus fill its lungs with an abundance of oxygen. Unfortunately, many dogs have to breathe the stale air of cities. Dogs will not exercise themselves fully in paddocks or runs, they will be apt to sit around waiting for the greater freedom offered by natural exercise outside their confines. Abundant daily exercise is needed for full digestion of a carnivorous diet. Also blood circulation is never normal in any dog denied its natural running freedom. Likewise, the organs of the body concerned with circulation—the lungs, heart, arteries, and veins—will diminish in strength with every passing year, until there will come the time when dogs will become semi-invalid years before their time, and no longer able to run tirelessly as the natural fox or wolf runs. The nervous system also becomes disordered, rendering the dog snappy or over-excited, or yapping or barking incessantly and without reason, typical of many kennel dogs. Also the coats of dogs lacking exercise are dull and often smell strongly because the blood which feeds the hair is sluggish.

DISCIPLINE. This is also of importance to total health. A wise observation: the bitch trains her whelps for nine weeks, then

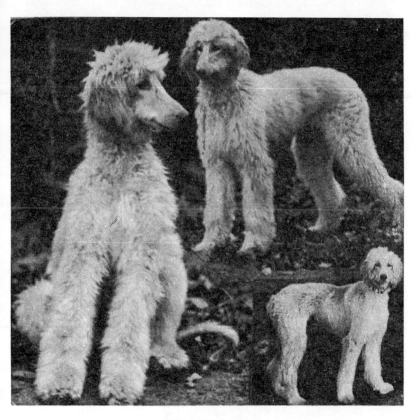

AFGHAN HOUND PUPPIES

Left: Turkuman Wild Bokhara Lily. *Upper right:* Turkuman Cinnamon Blossom; both bred by the author.
Lower right: Chota Nissim of Ringbank, bred by Doris Swann, Ringwood Afghans, Yorkshire. Nissim
was the most famous son of Turkuman Pomegranate and was later owned by Leo C. Wilson, the international judge. Nissim sired American Champion Turkuman Nissim's Laurel. Seven generations of
Turkuman Afghans were raised, were never vaccinated, never knew disease.

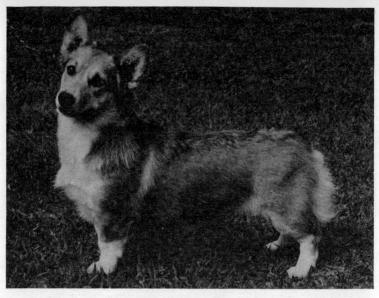

JESSICA'S PET OF BRAEDOON

Welsh Corgi. Mrs. Carol Irwin, Braedoon Kennels, 7A Great South Road, Manurewa, Auckland, New Zealand. This home-bred bitch puppy at eleven months was twice Best Puppy in Show All Breeds, and gained other top-flight show wins too numerous to mention. 'A picture of health from a N.R. litter of seven.' Mrs. Irwin is New Zealand Agent for Natural Rearing Products.

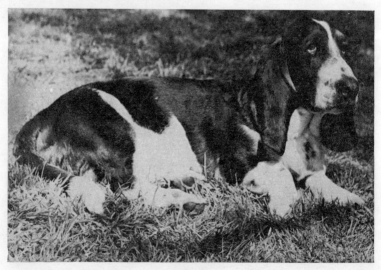

MAIDSMERE CAVALIER

Basset Hound Puppy. Mrs. Effie F. C. Clarke, Maidsmere, Finstall, Bromsgrove, Worcs. The wonderful bone and build of this tri-colour Basset Hound puppy speak for themselves. Mrs. Clarke is a keen follower of N.R. and is raising some splendid Bassets.

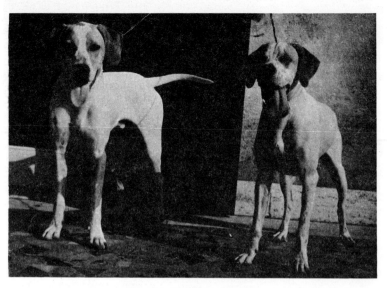

ROMER AND JULIETTE

Pointers. Alberico Boncompagni Ludovisi (Prince of Venosa), Roma Capannelle, Italy. Home-bred and N.R. reared by the Prince of Venosa, who also raises cattle by Nature methods, and who writes, 'They really are a credit to your tenets; beautifully built, never have experienced one day of either discomfort or poor appetite, nor been through any phase of "awkward looks" which is customary in young pointers. Once again your work is proved to be on the right path as far as animal husbandry is concerned.'

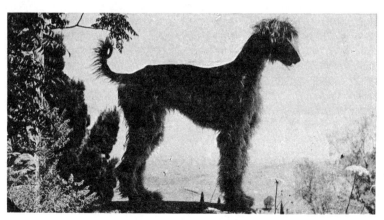

TURKUMAN WILD SEA HOLLY EL-JUDEA

Afghan hound. Juliette de Baïracli Levy, Tiberias, Israel. A rare junior silver bitch with dark grey shadings and bronze ear fringes. Possesses the best of the Turkuman blood-lines preserved by Juliette de Baïracli Levy's friend Cynthia Madigan, when travels made the breeding of Turkumans impossible for the author. Sea Holly is simply the best Afghan Juliette de Baïracli Levy has ever owned, both for type and intelligence. Blues and silvers predominate in her blood-lines. With her coat clipped for summer in Israel, the photo shows her beautiful lines. Photos of her are featured in many books. (*Photo: Rafik Bairacli*)

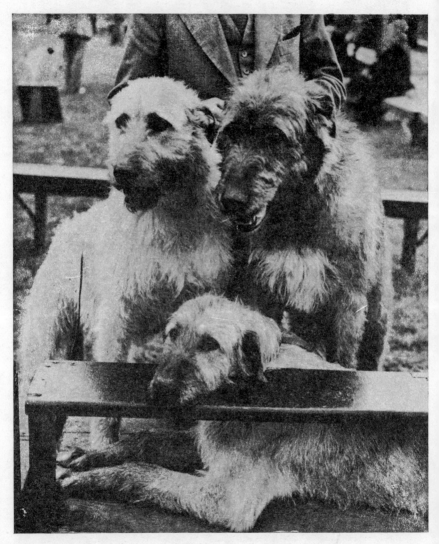

IRISH WOLFHOUND CHAMPIONS

Boreen of Ballykelly, Brangan of Ballykelly, and An Tostal of Ballykelly. Miss Sheelagh Seale, Ballykelly Kennels, Avoca, County Wicklow, Eire, a friend of the author, whose kennel was one of the first of the great kennels to follow N.R. These hounds are famed for their size and stamina, and are exhibited throughout Eire and England. (*Photo: Irish Independent Newspapers Ltd.*)

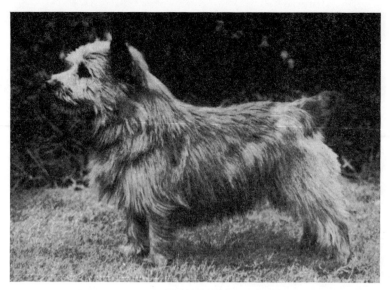

NORWICH TERRIER

Norwich Terrier. Mrs. E. H. Hardy, Quartzhill Kennels, Winscombe, Somerset; an enthusiastic follower of N.R. Mrs. Hardy (like the author) gives names of plants to all her famous Norwich terriers, and she has made many champions. (*Photo: Sally Anne Thompson*)

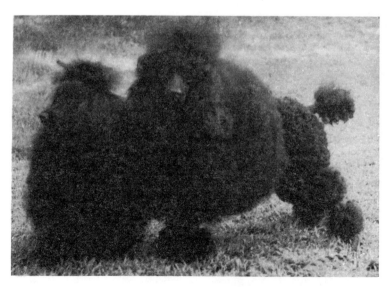

BLACK MINIATURE POODLES

Black Miniature Poodles. Mr. and Mrs. B. Heber-Percy, P.O. Box 38, Somerset West C.P., South Africa. Nine C.C.s between them and shown all over South Africa. Nature-reared and nature-fed, no inoculations or injections. (*Photo: Heber-Percy*)

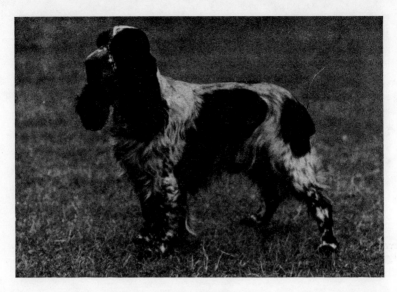

COCKER SPANIEL

Mrs. K. J. Gold (Fyer), Oxshott Kennels, Welwyn, Herts., an early pioneer of herbal treatment and N.R. in the canine world. She has helped many kennels to cure their sick dogs. Her own cockers are famed for health and type. (*Photo: C. M. Cooke*)

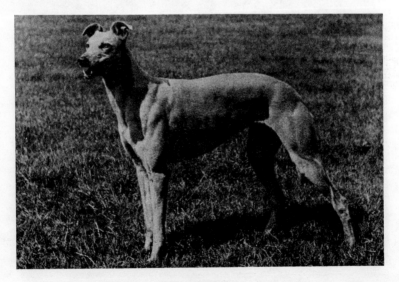

RACING GREYHOUND

Miss Peggy E. Brown, Headland Cottage, Harome, nr. Helmsley, Yorkshire. Nature-reared, this hound has won twenty-eight races and has been placed second twenty-four times. (*Photo: Bertram Unne*)

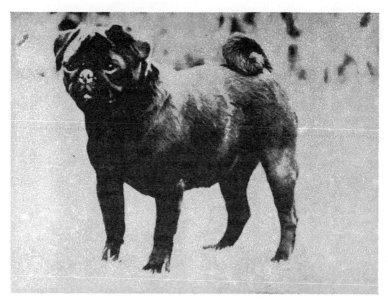

AMERICAN CHAMPION LOTUS OF LONGLANDS

Pug. Mrs. Bancroft-Wilson, Newton Abbot, Devonshire, bred and exported to the U.S.A. this famous dog. Considered a model pug. 'I have followed your herbal treatments from the beginning. Of invaluable help to my pugs, especially for whelping.' (*Photo: Walter Guiver*)

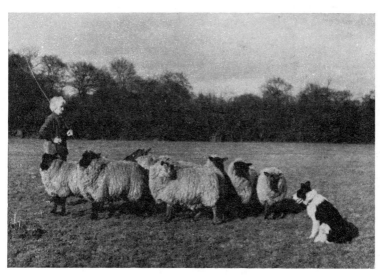

MEG

Border Collie. Mrs. Ivy Parry of International Sheepdog Trials fame, Ash Tree House, near Daventry, who believes in N.R. for her collies, sheep, and horses. Here seen working sheep. (*Photo: Raymond Brabbins*)

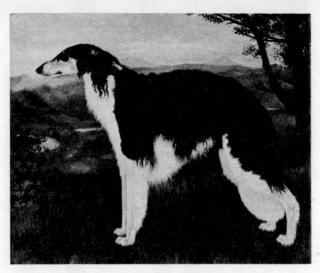

CHAMPION ZOMAHLI CHERMILA

Borzoi. Mrs. Lilian Pearson and Mr. Prior. Zomahli Kennels, Horsforth, Nr. Leeds, Yorkshire. This superb Borzoi dog created a breed record in England by winning twenty-two challenge certificates under twenty-two different judges. This kennel which believes in Nature Rearing has made thirteen Borzoi champions, and also won fame with the Saluki breed. (The author proudly owns and wears a silver rose antique bracelet given to her by Mrs. Pearson for help with Saluki health problems many years ago.)

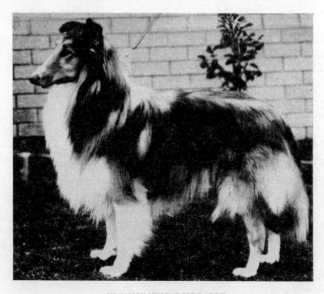

CHAMPION MYOENE BIG DADDY

Collie. Dr. and Mrs. E. W. Cramer, 43 Georges River Crescent, Oyster Bay, New South Wales, Australia. Top winning Collie. Working Dog Group. Top winner at Sydney Royal 1969 when only eighteen months. Has continued to win such awards as Best Exhibit at both Collie Club Show and Working Dog Shows. Many general Special Awards at All Breed shows. Sire of famed progeny. Mrs. Cramer is, and has been for many years, the Australian agent for Natural Rearing Products.

General Notes on Natural Rearing

man takes over. Human will-power concentrated on an animal's will, together with loving sympathy and strict daily routine, are the essentials for contented dogs. A young puppy should be trained from the time of weaning to the following requirements: (1) to respond to its own name; (2) to return when called; (3) to be cleanly in kennel habits; (4) not to steal or be greedy when feeding; (5) not to be quarrelsome with its fellow dogs; (6) to be friendly towards people but not to fawn; (7) not to whine or bark without real reason.

To bring out friendliness in kennel puppies, take them in turn into the home for visits.

A dog in its natural state would never soil its bed or yelp unceasingly without reason: it is man who has turned so many dogs into such unpleasant and dirty creatures.

Puppies should not be allowed to chew indiscriminately at anything they choose; they must be taught to exercise their teeth on suitable objects. The gypsies give roots for chewing to their greyhound or lurcher puppies, especially marshmallow roots, also cabbage stumps. I have found a twisted coil of rope gives good jaw exercise. Do not leave old bones lying around for mice and rats to contaminate or for flies to breed on.

Once the habit of house or kennel dirtying with urine or excreta has been acquired, the breaking of the habit is not easy. Put pepper on places where puppies have soiled; they will not return to the same place then. When puppies refuse to relieve themselves outdoors, to induce them to have a bowel action an infant-size suppository can be used for several times, or the fleshy stalk of a plant can be inserted into the anus. When the puppy has had a bowel action, it can then be much patted in praise and taken at once back into the house. Use the same words each time when the puppy is required to have a bowel action. Soon the puppy understands what is required of him and there is no further trouble. This is the simplest way to house-train a puppy.

INTERNAL CARE

This subject is mostly dealt with in the chapters on weaning, puppy diet, etc. However, it is my intention to include a few odd notes on puppy ailments and allied subjects not previously dealt with.

General Notes on Natural Rearing

COUGHING is a common symptom of distemper, or worms, or both. In olden times, distemper was described as 'the husk'. Immediate treatment consists of: fasting on honey-water, dosing with garlic or herbal tablets, or a strong brew of onions if the garlic is not available for immediate use. Elder blossom or berries, or sage, in a brew are also good. Temperature should be taken. Treatment details are given under Coughing, pages 112–13.

DEPRAVED APPETITE. This malady refers to the unhealthy habit of a puppy eating its own or other puppies' excreta. The eating of herbivorous droppings, cow pats, rabbit pellets, etc., is quite normal and healthful, and is only a typical canine search for extra herbal and mineral matter. But carnivorous excreta is highly toxic and harmful, and such a depraved eating habit must be checked. Worm infestation is a common cause, also boredom—especially lack of exercise. Canine faeces, in any case, should not be left lying on the ground to breed flies or spread parasitical worm ova; they should be removed promptly many times daily. Treatment consists of putting paraffin on the excreta to cause a repellent taste. There is also internal treatment, by increasing mineral intake with the feeding of twice the usual amount of daily seaweed powder given with the meat feed until the cure is complete. Supplying daily a large raw bone to chew at. Adding black treacle or molasses to the milk feed. It is also depraved appetite when a dog refuses raw meat and wants only cooked or canned food. Fast until *natural* food is accepted.

DIARRHOEA. (See pp. 68, 113–15)

DISCHARGING EYES. This may be a symptom of worms or distemper. Temperature of the puppy should be taken. The eyes should be bathed with a brew of common chamomile or fennel or balm leaves. A mixture of milk with the herbal brew is very effective; also witch-hazel: one part herbal brew, one-half teaspoon each of witch-hazel and milk to every two tablespoons of herb. The brew of elder blossom or chickweed or ground ivy are good, and when in season the juice of raw cucumbers, squeezed into the eyes.

DISTEMPER. (See Chapter 6.)

EATING FOREIGN BODIES. Puppies will eat wire, glass, tin, rubber, and other remarkable things often out of sheer playfulness. The best remedy is a meal of bread and milk, to mix around the foreign body, followed by a stiff dose of castor oil. For splinters of cooked bones—highly dangerous—lumps of cotton wool, not

General Notes on Natural Rearing

big enough to risk choking, can be rammed down the throat; a laxative dose of castor oil should follow later. (See also, Poison, as to method of inducing immediate vomiting.)

FITS, HYSTERIA. (See Chapter 6.) Immediate treatment is isolation in a quiet place. Stoppage of all food, fasting on honey-water diet. A daily laxative.

POISON. (See Chapter 6.) Puppies will eat such things as matches, poisoned vermin, and so on. A piece of washing-soda about the size of a small bean pushed down the throat will cause immediate vomiting. Larger breeds require several pieces of soda to produce vomiting.

RICKETS. This ailment is 100 per cent preventible, and is mostly due to unnatural rearing conditions. The predominant fault is unhealthy diet, especially the feeding of cooked and denatured foods. Additional fault is overcrowded kennel accommodation, lack of sunlight, and lack of contact with clean grassland; over-early weaning is also a cause.

Of what use is a dog without strong legs? And yet so many modern dogs possess malformed legs or shelly boned ones.

On sound puppy rearing—which means strong-boned stock—rests the whole future of a breed of dog. The health record of many of the best-known English and American breeds, at the present time, is not an enviable one; most breeds have quite a formidable list of hereditary ailments, specific ailments typifying the different breeds, the worst health records being among the oldest-established European breeds.

The one sure prescription for cure of rickets and general health improvement is to adopt fully natural rearing. The best herbal remedies for cure of rickets are: raw carrot, parsley, comfrey, and seaweed. Slippery-elm bark also should be used, as in the Natural Rearing gruel.

SICKNESS. Vomiting in the dog should always be encouraged; it is Nature's way of causing prompt internal cleansing. Vomiting following the eating of couch grass, mustard leaves, lichens, etc., is deliberate and cleansing and should be encouraged.

SORE FOOT PADS. (See Sore Pads, Chapter 6.)

STINGS. These are really external, but can be dealt with here. They are not dangerous except when on the tongue. Many puppies have a habit of snapping at wasps and bees. After removing the sting, the area should be rubbed immediately with a piece of

General Notes on Natural Rearing

washing-soda, dipped in water. This alkaline substance neutralizes the acid of the sting. A slice of raw onion or garlic can also be used, or raw lemon juice or witch-hazel—any of these applied to the sting area. Ammonia or white-wash (lime) are further safe aids diluted with three parts of water, but keep away from the eyes.

STOMACH SWELLING. Frequent swelling of the stomach following meals often indicates worms, for which treatment see Worms, Chapter 6. However, overfeeding may also be the root cause. 'Stonehenge' rightly says that 'art founded on experience' is required to fix the amount of food to give a growing puppy. The main test should be the eating up of all food greedily, no scouring, and no bloating. Puppies should still be active after each meal taken.

TEETHING. The first puppy teeth are milk teeth, appearing at four to five weeks of age, when the puppy is ready for solid foods. It should be a rule that no solids should be fed until the milk teeth first appear. These teeth eventually number twenty in the upper jaw, and twenty-two in the lower. They remain until the puppy is five to six months of age. No natural-reared puppy ever develops teething fits or other teething ailments. Sound and easily produced teeth are a natural heritage of healthy puppies. But for those breeders who are new to N.R., and have yet to produce N.R. stock, it should be emphasized that, should teething fits or other unnatural teething troubles occur, these should never be suppressed with chemicals. The puppy should be fasted for a day or two; dosed with a brew of skullcap or rosemary or sage, and the gums bathed twice daily with a brew of rosemary. N.R. diet, strictly followed, will then soon restore all to normal.

WORMS. (See Chapters 3 and 6.)

And now this puppy-rearing part is almost at an end, and it will be noted that, except for a few minor infant ailments, dealt with in an earlier chapter, the ailments are few—and yet most books on animal rearing devote three-quarters of the work to dealing with disease treatment. I have not just forgotten about disease! However, *if dog owners will truthfully and strictly follow the rulings and the teachings of this book they will achieve what I have achieved with my Afghan hounds in England, what Sir Albert Howard achieved with his cattle in India, and what numerous other breeders have achieved world-wide among their dogs: disease-free and disease-immune stock.*

General Notes on Natural Rearing

But perfection is not built overnight. And it took me many generations of careful rearing before I could get my Afghans up to a really high standard of health. Therefore, those breeders who do meet with disease must follow the curative treatments as given in Part Two of this book, in which all of the common canine ailments—both puppy and adult—are given in detail.

Breeders who experience sickness among their N.R. litters should not become discouraged. Nature is a slow worker: breeders are not going to get perfect, level, and unbroken health before a fifth generation of N.R. And when breeders have to use outside stud dogs they are undoing much of the good work (especially if such dogs are from inoculated stock). Quite positively, among my Afghan hound litters after the second generation I never had one day's illness. But the Afghan is a very 'natural' breed, which has not been spoiled by Western rearing methods, as yet. But, even so, occasional bouts of bowel looseness, disinclination for food, and so on, are quite a normal course of affairs in all infant rearing (children included). There must be an ebb and flow of health; toxins must accumulate from the very air (impure) that we breathe, especially in or near cities, alone, and from milk and other imperfect foods, even from cultivated vegetables which, unlike most wild ones, are often far from perfect and know disease themselves often enough; also think of today's prevalent low health standard of the animals upon whose flesh the domesticated dog must be fed. A short period of fasting and internal cleansing—usually a three-days' treatment—should soon normalize things, and will give improved health. When, of course, there is a deep infection, such as distemper, then treatment must be more prolonged; but, correctly treated by herbal methods, the disease will efficiently cleanse the organism and can only leave improved health. Disease awakens the latent healing powers of the body, tests them, and thereby strengthens them often enough. In rare cases disease treatment, by herbal medicine, may be prolonged into many months; many relapses may occur during treatment, but the final results will be total and permanent cure. Nature does not fail those who employ her diligently and faithfully.

Breeders having reared healthy puppies should then follow the principle of Mrs. F. E. Nuhn, Manakiki Kennels, of German Shepherds, Willoughby, Ohio, U.S.A. 'My adults and puppies are maintained in such marvellous hard condition on Natural Rearing,

General Notes on Natural Rearing

followed strictly as described in your books, that I am trying to educate my clientele to do as I do here or else they do not get a puppy!'

And when adding to their kennels, they should seek out N.R. stock in the manner of this Swiss doctor:

Dr. Alexander Schleidt, of Halisberg, Bernese Oberland, wrote to me: 'I am a faithful Swiss follower of your advice in your herbal books, which with your N.R. system has made my black and tan long-haired dachshunds so healthy, so full of pep, that they have become the terror of all neighbour dogs, foxes, badgers, hares, chamois, and deer, in the vicinity of our chalet! I now require a Pyrenean mountain dog as an extra guard, and since by long experience we know what wonderful results are obtained provided dogs are bred and kept according to your advice, I write to know of a kennel which follows the Natural Methods.'

Now and then I get negative reports from readers. They state that despite following the method given in this book, results have been bad. When I was first teaching Natural Rearing (and herbal veterinary medicine) to the canine world, I used to visit dissatisfied readers to find out what had gone wrong. Invariably I found they were not following my book at all, or very incompletely! They were failing in diet (usually giving cooked meat and a large proportion of canned foods): thus breaking the basic rule of Natural Rearing —the raw foods diet. The vital, daily, inclusion of chopped raw greens was omitted. Or there was almost no provision of running exercise. Or there was over-crowding. There was even use of vaccination in some cases. There was dosage with common chemical tonics—and so on.

I was always able to tell the dissatisfied with absolute truth, and with witnesses available wherever I had raised my own animals by my own method, in many lands, dogs, horses, goats, wild birds, bees, that they had all known excellent health, resistance to disease, and enjoyed long life. The good health on Natural Rearing, also included my two children, and the children of many other people. There, finally, I wrote a book on—Natural Rearing of Children, which Faber and Faber published in 1970.

Part Two

THE USE OF HERBS IN CANINE AILMENTS

5

Introduction to Herbal Medicine

In the following chapter of this Part Two, there will be found, in alphabetical order, the common canine ailments and the herbs that relieve and cure them. It is difficult for those who live in cities to go out and gather these herbs; they can be obtained dried if need be, but those who can collect their own are referred to the Appendix, where they are listed with their botanical names as well as a number of their popular (English) ones; so that with aid of any standard work on wild flowers one can identify the plants to be quite sure that the right plant has been found. The botanical name is the same for all countries, so that readers in Great Britain, the United States, Europe, and everywhere in the world should use a locally published book with illustrations as a guide. Most of the herbs used are common in England and America. For those who wish to use proprietary herbal products, some names and addresses of reliable firms are given in Chapter 8.

I have confined the ailments to the really common ones and to those that will respond to herbal treatment. I have not included in this book the vast number of canine diseases which are not readily curable and which are a direct result of long-term incorrect rearing —among them being tuberculosis, cancer, and other morbid growths, also other chronic ailments which afflict the canine race, and most of which, if correct rearing were followed—according to the laws of Nature—could certainly be avoided.

It might well be argued that if correct rearing methods were employed it surely then ought to be both possible and simple to avoid disease altogether. But it must be appreciated that in the domesticated conditions under which most dogs are kept, really natural rearing methods are very difficult to follow. There is, for

Introduction to Herbal Medicine

example, the flesh-foods question: the real flesh foods natural to the dog are mainly the smaller members of the animal kingdom, such as rabbits, hares, sheep, goats, etc., all of which are seldom available in the meat stores of big towns, and especially not as food for dogs. The meat that is commonly fed to dogs is, instead, usually old cow or horse, and in many cases the flesh being that of diseased animals which have died as a result of their sickness, or indirectly as a result of the dosing with chemical drugs. Other factors which can undermine the health, even of the strongest and most correctly reared dog, are inclement weather conditions, especially prolonged dampness of weather—the dog being a sunloving animal—and, further, infectious diseases carried by other dogs outside the breeder's own kennel, such as worms, skin parasites, and the several epidemic diseases. Then, furthermore, there are the hereditary ailments and the general inheritance of ill health which is the direct result of the unnatural rearing methods of the last eighty years or so, when men first began to commercialize dog breeding and introduce cheap rearing methods in place of the natural ones. Such methods include overcrowding in unhygienic kennels, breeding from weakly stock and, above all, unhealthy feeding. The standard diet used in breeding kennels up to seven or eight years ago—when the alarming state of canine health then forced breeders to adopt other feeding methods—was soaked white-flour biscuits with dried meat addition, the whole usually served up hot with greasy stock, and occasional lumps of cooked flesh and bones. Such an unnatural diet and 100 per cent cooked is still in common use today, with the difference that canned meat is now the unnatural way of feeding flesh to dogs and cats.

I have therefore confined the ailments mainly to those which are quite common, and which are likely to be met with, even in the best-managed kennels at times, especially because many conditions of the canine body which are described as diseases are in fact only cleansing efforts of the body, produced when the body has become internally unclean, or are simple glandular disturbances, to be found in young stock around the time of puberty. It is a natural fact that the adolescent period in young stock should be accompanied by minor body disturbances, just as the same period in children will often be accompanied by mild attacks of fevers, which, as in the case of canine distemper, are easily and readily cured, when *correctly* treated: but when incorrectly treated, by such

Introduction to Herbal Medicine

methods as chemical and serum therapy, can be turned into very serious conditions indeed, which well warrant the title of disease; and which can leave permanent sequelae, such as blindness, deafness, paralysis, nervous twitches, etc.

I have devoted much space to worm trouble, for more dogs are killed by dosing for worms than are ever killed by the worms themselves; and, further, severe suffering is frequently caused by the worm treatments in common use. Also, in this chapter will be found the internal cleansing treatment, which is a necessary and basic part not only of worm removal but of 90 per cent of canine ailments. (The treatment chart begins on page 99.) It may seem questionable that one treatment should form the basis for the cure of such a number of diverse canine ailments, but it must not be forgotten that Nature herself provides only one basic treatment, no matter what the body disorder is, be it broken limb or serious fever—and that is curative fasting and the attendant release of all the healing powers which are natural to every living thing, from a tree to a human being. Anyone who has studied the ways of wild animals cannot fail to have observed that in sickness the animal completely abstains from food, taking itself away into some quiet hiding place and there remaining until normal health state is restored to the body. It is then that the healed animal seeks out remedial herbs to complete the cure, and it is interesting to observe how the different animals show preferences for different herbs. For instance, the dog is very partial to couch grass, mustard leaves, and seaweed; the cat to couch grass and cat mint; the wild deer to bilberries and broom-tops; the hare to sow thistle; the cow to garlic leaves and watercress (when it can get the former!—for farmers ban it, unwisely).

I have given with the list of ailments instructions for the preparation of the herbal treatment. In every case the fresh-gathered herb should be used when possible, for it is only in the fresh state that all the wondrous healing powers contained in plant juices can be fully utilized; but, naturally, for the autumn and winter months it will be necessary to dry many of the herbs, although a number, such as rosemary, thyme, lavender, holly, and others are to a certain extent 'evergreen'. The herbs should be gathered when in full and fresh leaf, never when the leaf is fading; and for drying purposes a fine day is necessary, for if the herbs are gathered when rain- or dew-wet they will soon turn mouldy. To dry: they should

91

be spread out on the ground, on sheets of paper, where the sunlight can reach them, being frequently turned over to ensure complete drying. But if the sunlight is very strong, it is preferable to spread over the herbs a thin cotton cloth, especially cheesecloth, for very bright rays cause undue fading, making 'hay' instead of herbs! The whole subject is dealt with completely in my full-length practical herbal handbook—*Herbal Handbook for Farm and Stable*, published by the publishers of this present book.

The dried herbs should then be bunched and hung in a sunny or warm indoor position to finish the drying process; then they should be packed in cardboard boxes between sheets of paper (preferably greaseproof) or put into glass jars, which should be kept away from the light. In the case of complete absence of sunlight at a time when it is necessary to dry the herbs, which is not unknown in parts of the world during the herb-drying season in late summer, a lukewarm oven should be used for the drying. Herbs must be gathered fresh every year for drying, no matter how well they may have kept through the winter. Old herbs should not be retained; for that reason it is preferable for dog breeders to collect and dry their own herbs. In case of an emergency, dried herbs can be obtained from herbalists, but they may not be fresh and are almost always artificially dried, which destroys some of their value.

I can, however, guarantee that any herbal firm which I recommend will supply fresh, naturally dried herbs and preparations, and they are able to send them to overseas readers as well as those in Great Britain by post.

PREPARATION OF HERBS

STANDARD INFUSION. The standard infusion used throughout this book is made from one handful of the fresh herb (or two tablespoons dry herb), cut up small if the herb has large leaves, prepared with a pint of cold water. Cover well, then simmer until near boiling point, do not boil. Then stand, off the fire, to brew for four hours. Do not strain. Pour into a clean jar, covering this with paper—not waxed—or cotton cloth against dust, etc. Make a fresh infusion every three days or so.

The average dose (throughout this book a cocker spaniel-size dog is taken to represent average) is two level tablespoons of the infusion morning and night, and always at least thirty minutes

Introduction to Herbal Medicine

before a meal. For the smaller and larger breeds, decrease or increase the dose accordingly. Unlike chemical canine remedies, all herbal medicines are entirely harmless and therefore there is no fear of an overdose. That is why it is safe to give directions in handfuls, the need for extreme accuracy arises only when chemicals are used. Of course there are poisonous plants; but the herbalists should not deal in them. With the exception of opium poppy for urgent pain relief, they are unnecessary and dangerous, and I will not have my herbal work associated with them.

The best way of administering the infusions is from a medicine bottle with the correct dosage; the neck of the bottle is pressed into the near side of the dog's mouth and the bottle slowly emptied.

STRONG INFUSION. When stronger infusions are required, the shredded herbs should be placed in an enamel pan with one-half pint of *cold water* per handful of herbs (or more can be made at one time in proportion). Heat to boiling point, boil for no longer than three minutes, then set aside to brew for at least seven hours (it is preferable to leave overnight). Throughout the heating and steeping periods, keep tightly lidded to prevent escape of steam and volatile properties of herbs. After steeping, pour into a jar, without straining, and cover to exclude dust, etc. But allow entry of air.

Most herbs for canine use need this preparation, because their cellulose is not easily digested by carnivorous animals. Human beings, cattle, and horses can, of course, digest large quantities of raw herbs and obtain more easily their medicinal benefits. Dogs are exceptionally difficult to dose and must have their herbs very finely cut up or in powder form, either mixed into balls with honey and pushed down the throat, or well blended with their food. The former is to be preferred, as the bitterness of the herbs present may cause the dog to refuse the rest of the food.

I have evolved a method of giving herbs raw which has proved very effective. A herbal extract, very concentrated, may be given in a small dosage, no more than one tablespoonful twice daily for an average-size dog. To make the extract, squeeze a large handful of the fresh herbs into a ball, place on a good grater for vegetables, bruise herb by rubbing well on grater with flat of fingers. When herb is pulpy, put it on a square of cheesecloth or cotton and add an extracting medium (raw milk or carrot juice, both particularly absorbent), two tablespoons of raw unboiled milk or one medium-

Introduction to Herbal Medicine

size carrot. When liquid and herb pulp are mixed, wring and twist cloth strongly. The extract retains all vitamins and cosmic forces unspoiled, and the flavour is strong and aromatic, far more so than with the general hot-water extraction method.

PRACTICAL MEDICAL TREATMENTS

For the benefit of the novice, here is how to take a dog's temperature: Insert the mercury end of the thermometer in the anus (the opening of the lower bowel beneath the tail) so that all the mercury is covered. Keep the thermometer in that position for several minutes: then withdraw and read. Remember to shake the mercury well below the level of the normal temperature of 101·4° F. before inserting. ('Normal' is different for every creature. A special dog thermometer can be bought at a chemist's.) High fever is indicated by a temperature rise of 103° to 107° F. Wash the thermometer in cold water and pine fluid after use.

To give a suppository: Do not first use vaseline or glycerine as usually directed on the box wrapper; merely press the suppository into the anus and prevent the dog from expelling this for from three to five minutes.

To give an enema: a small bulb rectal syringe is required and about one and a half pints of warm water into which a teaspoon of witch hazel has been mixed (the witch hazel tones up the bowel walls); or lemon juice or tea-water can replace the witch hazel. Fill the syringe with the warm water and inject into the lower bowel slowly and steadily. Continue until all the fluid has entered the bowel, the animal's hind quarters being kept raised throughout. Then the dog will have a cleansing bowel evacuation. This type of enema does not take more than five minutes to carry out and is invaluable; as with herbal infusions, the quantity given is for an average dog, more or less fluid is required for larger or smaller breeds.

INTERNAL CLEANSING TREATMENT AND CHART

As the internal cleansing treatment chart, which I have evolved, forms the basis of most of the herbal cures for the ailments given in *Medicinal Herbs*, I am giving it in detail at the end of the chapter.

94

Introduction to Herbal Medicine

The chart was created especially for canine distemper cure, and therefore, except in cases of fever ailments, can be considerably shortened. For instance, for a short course of internal cleansing, merely a two-day fast followed by a further two-day milk-honey fluid diet would be necessary; a return to normal diet could then be made.

Special Note. Treatment must begin with a fast of at least two days on water or honey-water only. Two to three days is usually sufficient to cure a straightforward fever case. During fasting all the body powers released from food digestion are concentrated on elimination of internal toxins, and therefore chances of curing the ailments are made more favourable. Urgency of toxin elimination supplies the important reason for use of a daily laxative when fasting or on the fluid diet of milk and honey. During long fasts if there is no natural bowel action, a warm-water enema is given. Until the temperature is normal and steady at normal, fasting *must* be continued. To feed solid foods during a fever positively means complication of the ailment and often also means fatal results.

When people do not want to put their animals on a total fast, honey and fruit juices such as grape or apple can be given. Honey and grapes feed the body more completely than meat, etc., and are easily digested.

FASTING. In order to carry out with confidence this important part of the internal cleansing treatment, the principle of fasting must be understood. It is the natural instinct of all animals to fast when sick or wounded, because immediately all food is withheld, all the forces of the body are concentrated on fighting the disease or healing the wound, for the strength of the body is no longer being used up in the normal and continuous daily activity of food digestion, absorption, and elimination. Actually, when an animal is ill with fever, Nature discourages the intake of food by removing a desire for it and suspending senses of smell and taste: during acute fever, food digestion is checked almost totally.

If food is given forcibly at such times, severe bowel inflammation and thus diarrhoea are caused, and nerves also become inflamed. The chance, then, of the case making a satisfactory recovery is seriously diminished.

What actually happens during the fast? The body contrives to burn up the useless fat deposits, and until *all* fat is burnt up the vital tissues are left intact. As large amounts of body impurities are embedded in the fatty tissues of the average type of domestically reared dog, the body begins to be cleansed deeply, as the fat is oxidized; also the stomach and intestines, relieved of their usual tasks of dealing with food, can now concentrate on clearing away mucus deposits, worms and their ova, toxins, etc. Therefore the critical stage of the fever, which is usually prolonged in orthodox treatment, is speedily overcome in the natural cleansing-fasting treatment, and after three or four days' fast all danger is frequently over. If, however, the case under treatment is already in an advanced stage through the owner's failure to discover the early symptoms, and therefore the dog, though sick, having been allowed to feed on heavy foods when its temperature was raised above normal, a long fast is often necessary, and in some cases a three weeks' fast is required to restore the temperature to normal. It should be stated here that the dog's own inclination cannot always be relied upon. No sick wild animal will eat food, but in the domestic dog natural instinct has often long departed, and the urge of habit hunger and routine meal times will often cause a sick dog to partake of food; furthermore, a greedy desire for food when high fever is present is frequently a serious sign of deranged nerves.

It has been well proved that any animal can fast for three weeks (provided drinking-water is available) without the slightest distress. The fur-seal male (bull) fasts for three *months* during the breeding season. Also, when animals hibernate through the winter months, they are carrying out a partial fast. In order to understand more about fasting because of its importance in my herbal veterinary work, I have carried out several experimental fasts myself. The first three days are the most difficult, as the habit of desiring food at certain hours persists: but when those days are past, the brain begins to feel unusually clear and a feeling of extra well-being is experienced. It is this general feeling of well-being which helps a very sick animal to make its recovery from a disease. I have achieved many long fasts, including one of sixteen days and one of three weeks.

The main difficulty in teaching fasting to the inexperienced is the superstitious belief that a person or dog not having food daily will starve. They think that one or two days without food is the limit of a human or animal endurance. And yet the Yogis of India will fast for many weeks without thinking it an event of importance. The students of the famed philosopher Pythagoras were

Introduction to Herbal Medicine

required to fast their bodies for forty days before their brains were considered sufficiently purified to imbibe the profound teachings of this philosopher. The theory of rapid starvation is discredited when one considers that, in order to starve, the skeleton condition must first be reached, and an animal cannot starve while an ounce of fat still remains on its body. And considering that a fever case should be spending its time resting undisturbed in an even temperature, with access to as much fresh drinking-water as desired, very little expenditure of energy is needed and its normal fat supplies will last several weeks.

Dr. Herbert M. Shelton writes knowledgeably concerning fasting and the lesson to be learned from animals. 'Domestic cattle may often be found suffering from some chronic disease. Such animals invariably consume less food than the normal animal. Every farmer knows that when a cow, a horse, or hog, or sheep, etc., persistently refuses food, or day after day consumes much less than normally, there is something wrong with the animal.'

Dr. Felix Oswald states: 'Serious sickness prompts all animals to fast. Wounded deer will retire to some secluded den and starve for weeks together.'

Dr. Edwin Liek, a noted surgeon, endorses fasting, and observes that 'small children and animals, guided by an infallible instinct, limit to the utmost their intake of food if they are sick or injured'. He describes the instinctive fasting of three of his dogs. One was run over, suffering internal injuries and broken ribs; the second ate a quantity of rat poison; the third lost an eye in a fight. All three fasted and recovered, apart from eye replacement.

Professor Edmond Bordeaux Szekely has told me that once when his great hunting cat, Arriman, who used to catch and eat rattlesnakes, was bitten in the foot by one of those snakes, the cat allowed no one to touch him. He went to a swift-running stream, where he selected and ate quantities of a grass growing by it; he kept his injured foot deep in the water for one entire day and night with no other food. He fully recovered. Animals are usually their own best doctors.

Physiologists have persistently ignored those cases where dogs have voluntarily fasted for ten or twenty-eight or more days when suffering from broken bones or internal injuries. Here is an action invariably pursued by Nature which they persist in refusing to investigate. The enforced fasting of animals during modern war-

Introduction to Herbal Medicine

fare when trapped in bombed buildings, has given many remarkable examples, cases having survived after as long as one month without food *or* water. Then sheep have been buried for months in snowdrifts and have been rescued alive: but they have been able to eat the snow for water.

Those who have had no experience of fasting claim that it weakens the body. But the first weakness of fasting is merely due to habit hunger and passes after the first few days. Food does not give strength during fever. I have seen too many examples of the 'three-hourly feeds' orthodox treatment, which remove all doubt as to which treatment is correct, the natural or the unnatural. The feeding-during-fever cases are generally skeleton thin and foul-smelling internally, their bodies jerking with chorea, racked with fits, and many blinded with excessive eye discharges.

Then it is further often stated that without food during fever the blood is weakened. That such a statement is unscientific is demonstrated by the fact that laboratory tests of the blood of fasting cases, made before, during, and after the conclusion of the fast, show that the number of the vital red blood corpuscles is considerably *increased* by the animal having fasted.

I cannot over-emphasize that the giving of food to an animal with a high temperature is positively and undeniably the cause of most of the nervous complications found in canine distemper, for example. Out of the hundreds of fever cases sent to me for treatment, only a very few cases developed mental symptoms, and each of them had reached me in a very advanced stage of the disease; the damage to the nervous system had been caused already.

The good quality of the drinking-water is of utmost importance during long fasting, and in most large cities, where the water supply is heavily chlorinated, it is advisable to buy bottled spring water, usually obtainable from chemists. Do not buy unnatural distilled water or bottled water 'purified' by unnatural methods. Rain-water is good if collected in clean country air.

Of importance is the daily cleansing of the bowels. If diarrhoea is present or not, a daily laxative is still needed during fasting to cleanse away mucus and other impurities being loosened. Senna pods are best (for preparation, see Internal Cleansing Diet Chart). In lengthy fasting, give a rectal enema (see directions, page 94).

The fast must be continued while the temperature is around 102·6° F. or above, food not being permitted until the temperature has remained steady around 101·4° F. for at least four days. If the fever should return when the second, or feeding stage, of the treatment is in progress, this event being indicated by a sudden abrupt rise of temperature to around 103° F. or above, then the fast must be followed again. Such relapses are not common, but the fact that they do occur occasionally should not be ignored. Note that the normal temperature of young puppies is often 102° F., especially the excitable ones who have a normal temperature of around 102·8° F. It is seldom necessary to fast a young puppy longer than two to four days before a cure of fever symptoms is obtained.

Throughout the fasting stage pure honey can be given, and in exhaustion give juice of fresh grapes or apples or pomegranates. Two dessertspoonfuls at usual meal times, when food would have been given if the case was not being fasted, is an average dose for a medium-size dog.

Herbal tablets of powerful antiseptic herbs, with a garlic base, should be given morning and night, two three-grain tablets being an average dose each time. Their use is highly important. If these are not available, then rosemary herb, as sold in tins or packets at grocery stores, should be brewed by the standard method, and into this, when cold, should be crushed some garlic juice, using a juice extractor or mincing the garlic and pressing it through muslin —a small teaspoon of garlic to one dessertspoon of rosemary for an average-size dog. *Note:* Average size means spaniel (see page 92).

Internal Cleansing Diet Chart (*for Fever Cases*)

The amounts given here are for an average-size dog. Decrease or increase according to size of the individual breed.

First day. Three meals per day of tepid water only. One teaspoon of pure lemon juice can be added per meal. Do not use bottled or synthetic lemon juice.

Two herbal compound tablets or garlic plant, for internal disinfecting, morning and night throughout this treatment. Some form of laxative, preferably senna (two to two and one-half large senna pods, soaked seven hours in two tablespoons cold water, with a pinch of powdered ginger added, is average). Do not give oil laxatives. Give senna at night.

Second day. Repeat first day, including laxative at night.

Introduction to Herbal Medicine

Third day. Three meals per day of honey and water (one heaped teaspoon of honey to one cup of tepid water). Also fresh water to drink. Laxative.

Fourth day. Repeat third day. Laxative.

Fifth day. Repeat third day. Laxative.

Sixth day. Repeat third day. Provided the temperature is now normal, around 101·4° F., the honey-water can now be replaced by three small meals daily of unboiled cow's or goat's milk, preferably unpasteurized, of course, as heat treatment destroys the healing properties of milk. Pasteurized milk may have to be used if no other is available.

Now give Natural Rearing vegetable tablets, two tablets per day. If tablets are not available, give minced green salad vegetables, such as dandelion, watercress, turnip, and mustard greens, one dessertspoon at meal times. Suggested times for meals, 8 a.m., 12 noon, 6 p.m. Laxative to be discontinued.

Seventh day. Repeat sixth day.

Eighth day. Repeat sixth day, but alter evening meal by adding to the milk-honey one handful of flaked cereal, barley preferably; otherwise, use oats.

Ninth day. Repeat eighth day, increasing cereal to two handfuls.

Tenth day. Repeat eighth day, but now increase cereal to an ample feed. Sprinkle the cereal with powdered or flaked natural wheat germ, approximately one tablespoon. A few raisins, cut up small, can be added.

Eleventh day. Repeat tenth day.

Twelfth day. Cease 8 a.m. meal and replace midday meal with one cup of steamed fish plus a sprinkle of flaked oats and wheat germ.

Thirteenth day. Repeat twelfth day.

Fourteenth day. Repeat thirteenth day.

Fifteenth day. Repeat first day, i.e. water fast, to rest and re-cleanse the internal organs.

Sixteenth day. Repeat twelfth day, but now add other cereals to the barley-milk feed; preferably whole-grain oats, rye, etc. A little whole-grain bread or some whole-grain biscuits can be fed now.

The dog should now be ready to go on to the normal natural-rearing diet chart (see Chapter 1, page 43).

An important additional food is now the oxygen obtained only through outdoor running exercise.

Introduction to Herbal Medicine

Note. The carrying-out of the internal cleansing diet chart is left to the discretion of the person in charge of the sick dog or cat. It should always be remembered that the diet is dependent upon the temperature, and the presence of any fever should always be treated by fasting. Also great care must be taken in the ending of the fast. No more than stated quantities of solid foods given on the chart are permitted. To allow a dog to gorge itself after a long fast on fluids could have fatal results. The fasting must be ended carefully and gently, only very small amounts of solid foods being given for the first few days.

Fruit juices are permitted during fasting. But do not give orange or tomato, neither being beneficial foods for sick dogs.

6

Ailments and Their Treatments (in Alphabetical Order)

Note. For Standard Infusion and Strong Infusion, see instructions, Chapter 5, under Preparation of Herbs, p. 92. Therefore, unless otherwise stated, the amounts of all herbs prescribed in the treatments are: one handful of fresh or two tablespoons dry herbs to one pint of water.

ABRASION. Caused usually through biting at an itching part, especially in skin diseases, or can be caused through ill-fitting collar, or from an accident which tears off the hair.

Treatment. Make an infusion of young leaves of *blackberry* and apply externally twice daily; a little witch hazel extract can be added with advantage: one-quarter teaspoon witch hazel to every tablespoon of the blackberry infusion. *Elder* flowers and leaves or *rosemary* can be used instead. No greasy ointments should be used: such dressings soften the tissues and retard the cure.

ABSCESS. Found on any part of the body and commonly between the toes, where they are called interdigital cysts.

Treatment. Fomentations with *blackberry* or *elder* infusion, keeping the lotion hot during application. Do not add witch hazel now, as astringent is not required. An excellent poultice can be made by macerating three cloves of *garlic* root, or the heart of an *onion*. Stir this into two ounces of *castor* oil. Place the mixture in a small jar having a fairly loose cover, then place the jar in a pan of cold water to reach half-way up the jar, and bring the pan of cold water to a slow boil, heating the jar until the garlic or onion turns quite soft in the oil. Then wring out a piece of cotton in hot water, pour the hot lotion on to the hot cotton (but not too hot)

Ailments and Their Treatments

and bind over the abscess, using as a wrapping a piece of towelling that is dry and also hot.

An excellent alternative poultice is boiled *turnip* or *parsnip*, spread on cotton, as with the garlic-castor treatment.

ANAL GLANDS TROUBLE. Dogs rarely suffer from internal piles, but are quite commonly affected with a form of external piles known as anal glands trouble. The anus becomes swollen and surrounded with a number of small lumps which discharge blood when pressed. Haemorrhoids can also occur. Sufferers are usually overfed pets; also many of the toy breeds. The trouble would not occur if dogs were fed a natural diet which always included sufficient roughage.

Treatment. Dosing with a brew of *dandelion* (leaves and/or flowers); also, soak *fenugreek* seeds in warm water, two tablespoons to one cup or more, for twenty-four hours, then give the liquid as a drink, and feed the seeds mixed into the cereal feed. Give *linseed* tea, strong infusion; also apply the tea externally. In severe cases, make suppositories from pulped, raw *dock* leaves and insert in the anus. Also apply witch hazel.

ANAEMIA. Usually caused through incorrect diet or lack of sunlight, or constipation.

Treatment. Medicine of any of the black fruits, such as *bramble, bilberry, elderberry,* or *grape,* when in season, given crushed into the cereal feed or as a standard infusion. Two tablespoons of infusion for an average-size dog. Add a teaspoon of honey to every tablespoon of herbal infusion. When all the blackfruits are out of season, *nettle* can be used; this herb contains natural iron at its best, very different from chemical iron, which is constipating and aggravates anaemia. Feed also raw eggs, *seaweed,* molasses, *parsley.*

APPETITE, LOSS OF. Loss of appetite is an unfailing sign of toxic condition in the stomach or intestines, or both. Many dogs live almost their entire lives in such a state, picking at their food instead of devouring it in the manner of a healthy dog; they are described as 'bad-doers', but they are merely internally clogged and filthy, or they may be deprived of normal free-running exercise, essential to maintain good health.

Treatment. Internal dosing with an infusion of *peppermint,* using the flowers and small stalks in addition to the leaves, if available. *Cress* seed, sown out of doors or indoors and cultivated until a

103

Ailments and Their Treatments

plant of three inches high with parsley-like leaves is produced, and given finely shredded with the meat feed, is an excellent appetite restorer. Grated raw apple is also good. A course of internal cleansing, to purify the entire digestive tract, is an essential part of the treatment; the fasting period should be anywhere from three to seven days or until the dog shows a really keen desire for any food offered to it. Careful dieting on natural-rearing lines (see normal diet chart, Chapter 1) is a further essential, in order to keep the digestive tract clean and healthy once it has been cleansed through the fasting treatment. Whenever a dog leaves any food in the feeding-dish, that food should be removed immediately and the dog kept without until the next mealtime. Giving food snacks in between the two meals per day permitted is fatal to good appetite and sound health. Plenty of running exercise should also form a part of the treatment. Charcoal tablets are an excellent appetite restorative; also minced-up raw celery. *N.B.* Exception to the feeding rule is the greyhound breed. Afghans, salukis, etc., are often slow eaters; their meals have to stay with them several hours, sometimes overnight.

ARTHRITIS. This ailment once rare in the dog has become quite common. Joints often become knobby and gait stiffens. Damp, sunless rearing, also lack of adequate exercise, all encourage arthritis, even though an over-acid diet is the chief cause.

Treatment. Internal dosing with *rosemary* brew; also feed chopped, raw *parsley* and *comfrey* leaves mixed in with the meat. Boiled *nettles* are also curative. Externally massage the area with a lotion of four tablespoons olive oil, one part linseed oil, to which add half-teaspoon *eucalyptus* oil. *Sunflower* oil is also good, used in place of the linseed.

BAD BREATH. Very common in old dogs, but also in young dogs of the toy breeds, this is generally due to food decomposition and to constipation; in old dogs bad teeth may be responsible.

Treatment. Internal dosing with an infusion of *rosemary* leaves, flowers, or both; the mouth and teeth can also be washed with some of the infusion. A short course of internal cleansing is necessary, followed by corrective dieting. If dogs were fed correctly, according to the laws of Nature, bad breath would never occur, and dogs would keep their teeth in good condition up to the time of their death, no matter how great their age. Regular cleansing, fasting, and correct feeding are especially necessary in the rearing

Ailments and Their Treatments

of the toy breeds; their stomachs and intestines are so minute, regular 'resting' is essential, and what little food is fed to them must be of the highest possible quality; using rye as half of the cereal ration would benefit the toy breeds. In general, in bad breath, the inclusion in the diet of shredded dried fruits would benefit all breeds; dry fruits sweeten the stomach and digestive tract and are gently laxative. It is possible to obtain charcoal tablets from most chemists: they will purify the entire digestive tract.

BALDNESS. This trouble is especially prevalent among certain breeds, especially the dachshund, chow and pekinese breeds, and is referred to in later pages of this book, under the heading of Mange. However, there is another less serious state of baldness which affects many of the smooth-coated breeds, especially when they are in a state of low health; bitches after the rearing of a litter for which correct dietary preparation had not been made, distemper after-effects, nerve disorders, etc. The condition can be cleared up quickly through corrective diet and external herbal washes.

Treatment. A corrective raw-foods diet, especially rich in fresh raw meat, with a daily dosage of raw chopped *dandelion* leaves combined with the meat (the copper content of dandelion leaves being especially effective in the treatment). Exposure to all possible sunlight. Washes of an infusion of *rosemary* leaves or *marigold* flowers, both equally excellent. The bald areas should be bathed daily with the brew of rosemary or marigold. A brew made from *daffodil* leaves is an old gypsy remedy for baldness and falling hair. Rub the resultant liquid into the affected areas several times a day. *Castor oil* applied externally, well massaged into the bare areas, has proved excellent and is extra effective when a few drops of oil of *eucalyptus* are added.

BLADDER TROUBLES (*stone and gravel, also irritability and inflammation*). Bladder and kidney disorders are extremely common in the modern dog, the latter certainly being hereditary to a large extent, although they are also readily caused through the same factors responsible for the majority of canine ailments: incorrect and unnatural rearing.

Treatment. Internal dosing with an infusion of the root of *couch grass*; this infusion is prepared differently from the standard method, the herb having to be simmered a full quarter-hour in the water. First, well bruise the root, then take two ounces of the root over which pour three-quarters of a pint of boiling water, simmer gently until only a half pint of the liquid remains; then brew and prepare in the usual way; couch-grass root possesses remarkable stone-dissolving properties.

Another excellent remedy is young *birch* leaves, infused in the standard way. A course of internal cleansing is recommended; and in the diet the addition of very finely shredded parsley and carrot added to the meat feed; the use of barley in place of the usual wheat cereal is very helpful (the barley must be whole grain, never 'pearl' or 'patent' barley, both being unnatural acid-producing foods). Pure honey gives remarkable aid and relief in bladder and kidney disorders, and is best given with the cereal feed. Operations for the removal of stone should never be resorted to until natural treatment has been given a thorough trial. Remarkable results have been obtained in the treatment of bladder and kidney disorders by the above method. The Rivaway Kennels, Beeston, Nottinghamshire, report: 'We had a Chow dog very ill with kidney trouble; the veterinary surgeon said he was a hopeless case, incurable. That is more than eighteen months ago; he is now a most beautiful dog (his photograph is in *Our Dogs Annual*, 1945). We gave him parsley water three times a day, and milk and barley water sweetened with honey. When his appetite came back, chopped parsley was added to his feed. He still has parsley and so do all the others.'

BLEEDING, OF WOUNDS. When there is a great amount of bleeding from a wound, the blood outflow should be controlled and the torn flesh soothed by the application of a healing herb infusion. In all but the very deep-seated wounds there should be no bandaging, for the action of the dog's tongue in keeping the wound moist and breaking up the pus formations is alone a most remarkable healing process, and bandaging would prevent the dog from making use of it. The formation of pus should never cause worry; that is Nature's own method of keeping the wound open and moist, for if a wound were to become sealed up at too early a stage in the healing process, any external impurities which may have found their way into the body tissue at the time of the wounding are then encouraged to set up poisoning, which may prove serious enough to cause death. In very deep-seated wounds the method of the great Spanish surgeon, Trueta, as practised with

Ailments and Their Treatments

such success in the Spanish Civil War, should be followed. The wound should be laid freely open, all damaged tissue cut cleanly away so that the wound is left well open. Then pack the wound round with damp cotton wool and immobilize by making a loosely fitting plaster-of-Paris jacket to cover the injured part; note carefully the instruction 'loosely fitting'. The deep wound is then left to the healing powers of Nature; the formation of pus keeps the wound open and moist until the internal tissues are well healed.

How very different from the artificial methods of chemical medicine, so popular until Surgeon Trueta's remarkable results in wound healing caused his method to be adopted by large numbers of doctors in place of the orthodox one, with its harmful dry gauze placed over the raw wounds, the frequent scraping away of all pus formations, and the application of chemical disinfectants: the Trueta method has revealed the harm done in medicine, in my opinion, by Pasteur's friend, Joseph Lister, the pioneer of chemical disinfectant wound dressings.

Treatment. Herbal treatment to control the flow of blood from a severe wound, and to soothe and cleanse the injured tissues, is provided by a strong infusion of *rosemary* or the *meadowsweet* plant, both flowers and leaves being used, or hyssop. The infusion can be used both externally and internally; if given internally it strengthens the tissue-repairing powers of the body. If the wound is very deep, and it is therefore necessary to use the Trueta method, an excellent natural dressing for packing around the wound beneath the plaster covering is *sphagnum moss*. This moss is a remarkable herb; it grows in damp places, in many parts of the world. The chief property of sphagnum moss is its natural iodine content. (It would not be out of place here to warn against the use of artificial chemical iodine, once the most-boosted wound and bruise treatment of the orthodox medical profession. In the words of one of the great pioneers of natural healing, Dr. Lindlahr, 'the action of chemical iodine on living tissue is that of a mummifying agent, and prevents all normal healing, while encouraging the growth of excessively coarse scar tissue'. The same can be said for almost all of the chemical disinfectants.) Another important treatment rule is: if the wounds are severe, and loss of blood considerable, a fast of one to several days is very necessary: most animals will voluntarily refrain from eating when severely wounded. At such times all of the internal forces of the body are required for cleansing,

107

Ailments and Their Treatments

repair, and healing: they must not be wasted upon food digestion. Dosage with the leaf-extract tablets is most beneficial. For this green 'blood' of plant leaves does build red corpuscles and makes new blood in a far more natural way than transfusions of animal blood—as well as having none of the toxins that such blood must invariably contain.

Miss Sheelagh Seale, of the Ballykelly Irish Wolfhounds and Deerhounds, Avoca, Eire, reported the rapid recovery from severe wounds of a deerhound bitch. The bitch was badly bitten in a fight, and it was thought that she would die of her wounds. To quote Miss Seale: 'When the vet left after seeing her the first time, he said that my only hope to pull her through was sulphonamide drugs. The sulphonamides, of course, were *not* given. And when the vet came five days later the herbal treatment had produced the usual great results, and he was surprised to find the bitch so well, and all her wounds quite clean and healing up. The bitch has quite recovered now.'

On my world travels I have usually had an Afghan hound with me as a guard. Being swift-running and wild-natured dogs, they have had their share of physical accidents, especially deep wounds from sharp-pointed desert vegetation, sharp rocks, etc. I have never stitched any of their wounds, despite some of them being deep enough to insert a hand fully inside. I have only relied on the healing and antiseptic powers of *rosemary* as a wound lotion (and, when this was not obtainable, using the more common *plantain*). I have also healed the torn udders of cows, leaking milk badly, by using rosemary for bathing, and plugging wounds with witch hazel on cotton, and also with clean (not dusty) cobwebs—spiderwebs.

BREAST TUMOURS (*also other tumours*). Tumours in the milk glands area sometimes develop in bitches, and can be caused by blows, or merely from general ill health. Disordered glandular functions and constipation are also common causes, and an internal cleansing treatment, using the very solvent remedy *grape* juice, will often effect a cure. The tendrils and leaves of *grape* vine (from unsprayed vines), also fresh grape juice, have been used very effectively by the Arabs as an internal and external cure for tumours. The Mexican peasants use *nopal cactus* leaves, freed from prickles, in a way similar to the grape cure. *Violet* leaves have won fame with powers of dissolving tumorous and other growths.

108

Ailments and Their Treatments

There is recorded the case of Lady Margaret Marsham, whose throat was completely blocked by a malignant growth, and which growth was entirely dissolved through the use of violet leaves. The violet-leaf infusion should both be given internally—two tablespoons morning and night—and applied externally—massaging the area of the tumour with the infusion on rising and retiring. *Red clover*, the leaves and flowers, or merely the leaves, can replace the violet leaves for both internal and external use when there is difficulty in obtaining the latter. Garlic and turnip also dissolve tumours.

In severe cases, poultices made from fresh *goose grass* and applied to the affected area, are also very helpful. (The goose grass, like sphagnum moss, is rich in natural iodine.) Since the earlier editions of *Medicinal Herbs*, I have been lent back copies of that excellent journal, *The Countryman*, in which the effect of violet brew was discussed in detail in the correspondence columns of the Autumn 1941, and Spring 1942 numbers. Among much interesting information given, is the fact that the native doctors of Puerto Rico use a local violet (*viola odorata*) to cure mild cancer of the stomach. Tincture of violet is now in use in leading London hospitals. The Turks recommend large quantities of *watercress*, to be eaten daily, and cures have been achieved by this simple treatment.

BROKEN BONES. (See Limbs, Fractures of.)

BRONCHITIS. (See Pneumonia.)

BURNS. (See Scalds.)

CANCER. (See also Breast Tumours.) This terrible, killing disease was in former times almost unknown to the dog and the other carnivores. As chances of cure, even with herbs, are very slight, I am not going to suggest a herbal cure to prolong a disease usually so painful, and fatal. Cancer is alarmingly on the increase among domestic dogs and cats. Thousands of these loyal animals die every year after great suffering. *Prevention* depends upon natural rearing on pure natural foods similar to what the carnivores and felines eat in the wild; also provision of sufficient exercise.

CANKER. Canker of the ear is common to the domestic dog, especially to the breeds with long ear flaps which exclude air. One form of canker can be treated only by surgery; this is when heredity over-narrows the ear passage, excluding all normal air; a false air duct has then to be made by surgery. Long ears, especially, should be cleansed daily with standard rosemary infusion, three parts, and one part witch hazel extract. Keep inner-ear flaps clean, using diluted witch hazel.

Treatment. Numerous cases have been cured by simple use of raw *lemon* juice, one-half teaspoon of the juice diluted with one and one-half dessertspoons warm water. If the canker is simple, and not caused by an ear parasite, it will merely be necessary to cleanse the ears daily, internally, with an infusion of *horehound*, or one made from equal quantities of *violet* leaves and *wild poppy* leaves. The ears can then be further cleansed with witch hazel extract to remove the waxy deposits, and finally dusted over with finely powdered oatmeal; or the witch hazel could be used with the horehound or violet-poppy infusion, i.e. to one teaspoon of the infusion, four drops of witch hazel may be added. To cleanse the ears: twist a swab of cotton wool around the end of a pair of long tweezers, dip into the lotion, and very gently clean out the ear, frequently changing the cotton wool; about one level teaspoon of the lotion can then be dropped into each ear every morning, and well massaged; the ear being cleaned out with the tweezers and *dry* cotton wool in the evening. I have seen this lotion cure ears which were entirely blocked with the dark matter found in neglected or incorrectly treated ear canker.

In the form of canker caused by a small insect parasite, some insecticidal agent must be used. I can recommend with confidence my formula 100 per cent herbal insecticide powder, made into a liquid with hot water. One teaspoon of the herb makes a cupful of lotion. Use nightly. A few drops of eucalyptus oil can be added to sufficient lotion to cleanse both ears. (From N.R. Products, Manchester.)

N.B. It must be remembered that the ears are highly sensitive organs, and therefore the cleansing treatment must always be extremely careful and gentle; there should be no poking or prodding.

A short course of internal cleansing would improve the general health of the dog, which is often impaired when canker is present. An infusion of *garden thyme* can also be given internally as a tonic, and will thus soothe the inflamed nerves of the ear and head.

Mrs. N. Howard, the Chastletown gun-dog breeder, Wolverhampton, wrote me concerning two springer spaniel stud dogs which had been suffering for a long time from very severe ear canker, which had been unsuccessfully treated by three different

Ailments and Their Treatments

veterinary surgeons. In her first letter, Mrs. Howard told me that the condition of the dogs' ears was so bad she thought that she would have to have them both destroyed. However, internal cleansing was suggested to her, in addition to the usual external treatment with herbs. The ears of both dogs were entirely cured and the dogs themselves became very healthy.

Mrs. Leslie Harrison, of Tarporley, Cheshire, famous for her pedigree goats and borzois, reported to me: 'A spaniel condemned by a foremost North-of-England vet as having incurable ear canker, is now rising thirteen years and completely cured by your herbal treatment and so full of life it is wonderful to see him.'

CATARACT AND EYE ULCERS AND AILMENTS. Vitamin A is an important preventive of eye infections. To ensure its presence in the daily diet, raw, green, minced vegetables should be given. Vitamin A is also present in animal fats such as unrefined cod-liver oil, halibut oil, meat fats, nut fats, and whole, raw milk. Further, in raw and cooked carrots and sunlight.

Treatment. Bathing the eye with an infusion of the leaves and flowers of the *greater celandine*, favourite eye remedy of the famed herbalist of ancient times, Culpeper. The eyes should be bathed twice daily with the celandine infusion which is to be used externally only. A course of internal cleansing should also be followed, to strengthen the whole body and thus the eyes also.

A strong infusion of flowers of *rue* or leaves of *sage* is used by Spanish peasants with much success. Use the same way as greater celandine. A standard infusion of either *rosemary*, *chickweed*, *mallow* flowers, or *dock* leaves—all are good for inflamed eyes, as also is raw *cucumber* juice squeezed into the eyes, and, further, cold Indian or China *tea* can be used with benefit for bathing them.

CHOREA. Although nearly always a sequela of wrongly treated distemper, chorea sometimes occurs as a separate ailment. It is one of the most readily curable of the canine nervous ailments, the treatment given here having produced excellent results, healing many cases condemned as incurable by orthodox treatment.

Treatment. An infusion of *skullcap* herb, the whole plant. Two tablespoons three times daily. Other internal chorea aids are: *rosemary*, *peony* root, *vervain*, *cayenne* pepper (this pepper given in gelatine capsules, one-quarter teaspoon per capsule, morning and night).

For external treatment, make an infusion of *lavender*, *marjoram*,

111

or *thyme*, or an infusion of all three; apply hot to the twitching areas. Give a course of internal cleansing treatment as a general nerve tonic. Feed as an extra, minced *lettuce* leaves and garden *mint*, both sedative to the nerves, also *grape* juice, fresh or bottled.

CONSTIPATION. Just as correct diet is the only preventive of constipation, so likewise corrective dieting is the only cure for the ailment. No amount of dosing with chemical laxatives will effect a cure: such drastic dosing will only aggravate the trouble by weakening yet further the intestinal muscles, the healthy condition of which is essential for the regular and complete evacuation of waste matter from the body. In constipation, the toxins of the waste matter of the body, instead of being expelled daily through the bowel, are retained in the body and absorbed back into the blood-stream. It therefore cannot be wondered at that constipation is the root cause of a large number of canine ailments, from the lesser ones, such as eczema, to the acute ailments, such as cancer of the bowels, now becoming a common complaint.

Treatment. As I have already said, the only curative treatment for constipation is through corrective diet, which will remove blocking toxic accumulations from the bowels, and will also restore to the intestinal muscles that natural strength which is necessary for the moving of the food residues down the bowel, and the complete expulsion of the bowel contents through the anus twice, or at least once, daily. The finest natural correctives of constipation, even in the case of the carnivorous dog, are fruits. Many dogs, if taught from puppyhood, will freely eat dried fruits with their cereal feed. Suitable dried fruits are figs, dates, raisins, and prunes—prunes being especially beneficial. Many dogs will eat fresh fruits and berries; they should be encouraged. Likewise, let them eat excreta of grass-fed animals. (See also notes on senna-pod laxatives, p. 99.)

COUGHING. Coughing in dogs is generally a symptom of some health disorders, from distemper to worms. The old-fashioned name for distemper was 'the husk'. (See Worms and Distemper.)

But when the cough is a result purely of an irritation of the mucous membrane of the throat or the upper parts of the alimentary canal, or disorders of the lungs, then local internal and external treatment will give relief.

Treatment. Make a strong infusion of *liquorice* root, using one tablespoon of the root or a one-ounce piece of the solid juice. Add

Ailments and Their Treatments

one pint of cold water and bring to the boil. Add one teaspoon of honey to each tablespoon of the liquorice brew. Give two table-spoons before meals. *Blackberry* leaves, *elder* blossom, *thyme*, the whole plant—all are good cough remedies, made in standard in-fusions. Also *black-currant* jam, stirring one tablespoon of the jam into a cupful of water: add honey.

Externally, friction the throat and chest with oil of *eucalyptus*, one teaspoon dissolved in one cup of warmed *olive* oil. Keep the area covered with heated towelling.

DENTITION (FAULTY) is a modern ailment. Normal tooth quota is deficient, usually it is the premolar teeth, one or two missing, usually in the lower jaw. This causes a great gap in the mouth, and food cannot be dealt with properly.

Treatment. Man cannot give the dog artificial teeth! The only remedy is prevention through a natural diet of whole foods.

DIABETES. This disease was a rare ailment of the dog until recent years, but it has now become quite a common one, in the same way that cancer has increased from rare to common. This incidence of canine diabetes is a severe warning against the folly of artificial diet; against the can of processed meat and the fancy carton of highly processed cereal known as 'dog biscuit'. Diabetes can also be caused by shock. There is also the insidious form of shock inflicted upon the sensitive canine body by repeated vaccina-tions of all kinds common to the modern dog. Veterinary diagnosis of blood and urine is necessary to detect diabetes.

Treatment. This requires a preliminary careful fasting, following the internal cleansing treatment, followed by the usual N.R. diet. Avoid the use of insulin; corrective diet is a far safer way of controlling and, in many cases, curing this disease. The cereal should be restricted, using *rye* in the N.R. diet, and this can be purchased from most grocery stores as a crisp bread. Use also as a cereal substitute *carrots*, either raw, grated, or lightly cooked. Carrots themselves, although often forbidden to diabetic cases, contain a natural-type insulin and are therefore really beneficial; so are Jerusalem artichokes. Medicines are powdered *oak* bark, a brew from shaved olive roots or from olive leaves, one teaspoon daily. Give also a daily dose of herbal antiseptic tablets.

DIARRHOEA. This is not usually a separate ailment, it is more often a symptom of some other internal disorder, such as gastritis, brought on by over-eating or through incorrect diet or the irritant

113

properties of chemical preservatives present in most processed foods. Presence of masses of worms in the digestive tract, or as a symptom of distemper or other fever ailments, can cause diarrhoea. Correctly treated, diarrhoea is easy to cure and often proves beneficial to the later health of the dog as it can serve as Nature's method of removing a dangerous accumulation of toxic matter in the body. Therefore in herbal medicine, treatment of diarrhoea is opposite to orthodox. The latter aims at immediate checking of the bowel flow by use of starchy foods or blocking preparations of the kaolin class. Herbal treatment encourages bowel flow by the use of vegetable laxatives such as *senna*, and juices of *figs* and other laxative fruits.

Treatment. All members of the *onion-garlic* family, also *lemon* juice, are specific remedies for diarrhoea, as they sweeten and soothe as well as disinfect the entire digestive tract. Fasting is essential in diarrhoea, for it is useless to burden the body with food of any kind at a time when all of the body energies are required for the removal of waste matter from the digestive tract. Food given at such times will merely ferment and further burden the sick animal. The fasting, apart from the giving of honey-lemon juice and herbal tablets containing garlic, should be maintained very strictly until all putrid odour and bad colour leave the bowel flow, then honey can be given both as food and healing agent. *Apple* juice is very healing in diarrhoea and can usually be given with benefit after the first forty-eight hours of the attack. (Now see the Internal Cleansing Diet Chart, Chapter 5, for introducing milk and cereals, especially tree-barks flour, which acts as an internal poultice, not blocking the digestive tract, but soothing inflamed areas with its vegetable jelly as well as nourishing the body.)

I have a typical report from Mrs. J. Kennedy, of Evershot, Dorset, concerning a Pekinese puppy which had had intermittent diarrhoea for three *months* and had been on orthodox veterinary treatment throughout that time with no success. The herbal treatment and use of my tree-barks food cured the puppy within one *week*, and there has been no return of the ailment. This same herbal cure has also won fame in the treatment of scouring sheep and lambs and has even cured many cases of the dreaded 'black scour' of sheep.

I recently used the food at the Dr. Lytton-Bernard Ranch, Guadalajara, Mexico, on a wild raccoon cub, deprived of its mother and fading from scour. The raccoon grew into a healthy adult.

I again used the food with good success, when I was in charge of Professor Szekely's goats in Tecate, Mexico, for treatment of weakly kids and in hand-rearing kids. And whilst working on this new edition of my first canine book I cured two orphaned hawks of chronic diarrhoea (photograph of one hawk is in this book).

DISTEMPER. Formerly I wrote a one-hundred-page book on the prevention and cure of canine distemper. This was included in its entirety in *The Complete Herbal Book for the Dog*. I later condensed this for the American edition, which is now replacing the English edition also in England, but I shall cover the subject sufficiently herein. The herbal treatment has already effected cures in kennels in the United States, speedily and completely, as it likewise has in numerous other countries of the world where it has been used.

Distemper in dogs is prevalent in most countries where the domestic dog is bred and dates back to the earliest centuries, and yet the cause of the disease has never been proved. Canine distemper is described in most veterinary medicine books as being a virulent, highly contagious ailment which is frequently accompanied by serious nervous complications. That is the orthodox description, resulting from unnatural treatments with sera, chemical drugs, and incorrect invalid diet. For my part, using simple herbal treatment, including fasting, I have found distemper easy to treat, speedy to cure, and devoid of any after complications. Testimonials world-wide, written in many languages, will uphold this statement.

That many breeders who have had entire kennels wiped out by canine distemper, and many owners who have lost their pets overfrequently from distemper, are seeking the herbal treatment has been proved by the large sales of this herbal book in the countries in which it has been published: England, Switzerland, Germany, Holland, U.S.A. In Switzerland it is veterinary surgeons who have translated my herbal books into Swiss-German.

The veterinary profession in most countries generally accepts nervous disorders as a usual accompaniment of distemper. And yet, out of the some thousand cases of this disease that I have treated, less than a dozen have developed nervous disorders, and in every one of those dogs the disease had been in a highly advanced

Ailments and Their Treatments

stage before coming to me for treatment. I have never had a case develop either chorea or paralysis. What, then, can the reason be for nervous disorders being prevalent in one treatment and absent following a different one? I am convinced, and have proved countless times, that the main cause of nervous complications is the unnatural practice of giving food to invalid dogs when high fever is present, i.e. temperature around or above 103° F. During fever all the normal processes of digestion are suspended, all of the body forces being concentrated on fighting the bacteria which are causing the fever condition; food given at such a time poisons the entire system and seriously impairs the animal's power to conquer disease. In most cases the dog will put up a frantic struggle against the forced feeding, but occasionally, nervousness caused by the fever will induce a dog to eat up all food that is given to it. When, as frequently happens, forced feeding through the mouth proves impossible because of the dog's struggle against this, the hypodermic syringe is used, and such unnatural substances as brandy, salines, and even blood are injected into the animal's fevered body. If a dog does recover from such treatment, he is usually left permanently nervous, in poor condition, and very susceptible to skin diseases, the normal health balance of the body having been destroyed permanently.

Then there is the further unnatural treatment of serum injections, the antibodies in the serum being supposed to aid the blood corpuscles in fighting the bacteria causing the disease. These shock injections into a disease-weakened body will often abate the cleansing processes of the case, and mucus discharges will cease abruptly; the temperature drops to normal and the animal is considered cured; whereas, in truth, the ailment has merely been suppressed, driven deeper within the body. After a week or so, it is common for the temperature of the serum-cured case to soar up again, and then invariably nervous disorders swiftly follow violent fits or paralysis. These symptoms are in turn suppressed by sedatives, and the dog then indeed passes beyond possibility of cure, and usually has to be destroyed. Nervous disorders (see Nervousness) can be cured by herbs, but they have proved difficult to cure when resulting from the unnatural treatment described above.

Symptoms of distemper are typical and easy to recognize. 'The husk', its old-fashioned name, alluded to the persistent, dry cough usually present in this disease. (Yet in some cases there is no cough

Ailments and Their Treatments

at all.) Beads of pus occur at the corners of the eyes, the nose is hot and dry. As the disease progresses the eye discharge becomes copious and there is also similar discharge from the nostrils. The mouth smells fetid, the eyes turn very bloodshot, and often diarrhoea is present. The temperature next rises rapidly, and with this rise the dog becomes very listless and troubled and seeks a dark place in which to hide itself. Food is refused and there is often much shivering.

Treatment. The dog must be fasted immediately (see Internal Cleansing Diet, Chapter 5). He must be isolated in a quiet, warm place, with a window sufficiently open to admit fresh air, day and night, oxygen being very important in this disease, or lung complications will develop. If the dog is being treated in a kennel, there should be a deep hay or straw bed provided and, again, ample fresh air. Herbal antiseptic tablets should be given night and morning, or simpler home-made pills from finely grated raw *garlic*, mixed with honey and a very little wheaten or other flour, to bind the mixture. The mouth and teeth should be cleansed morning and night, using very diluted *lemon* juice, one teaspoon of the pure juice (not synthetic) to two dessertspoons of water. It is advantageous if the dog also swallows some of this lemon water. Give several tablespoons each morning. Eyes and nose should be cleansed of mucus at least three times daily, using cotton swabs dipped into an infusion of any one, or a mixture, of the following herbs: *rosemary, elder flowers, chickweed, speedwell, balm.*

Any soreness of nostrils or eyes should be treated with an application of pure *almond* oil.

Honey-water should be given. If the dog will not take this, then give plain water and roll thick honey into pieces and push down the throat at what would have been meal-times if the case were not fasting. Honey does not tax the digestion in any way; being pre-digested by the bees when in the hive, it is absorbed immediately into the blood-stream.

When the fever has ended, the dog can be immediately taken off the internal cleansing treatment, and the natural-rearing diet followed instead. During the treatment the dog should be taken outdoors sufficient times to relieve itself. The movement of limbs is beneficial, also the change of air.

If diarrhoea persists even after the fever has ended, add tree-barks preparation to the milk. This flour will soothe the digestive

117

tract as well as provide nutritious yet light food. Sprinkle a small half teaspoon of powdered *cinnamon* to every cupful of tree-barks flour.

If all food is persistently refused by the dog even after temperature has been normal for some time, a return of the fever can be expected soon, and the case must be fasted a further period until fever subsides.

Throughout distemper treatment, for at least three weeks or more, the dog's temperature should be taken night and morning. Use a clinical thermometer of the 'stub', not finely pointed, kind. The whole dietary régime of the case is dependent upon the temperature readings.

Suggested times for honey, etc., are: 8 a.m., 12 noon, and 7 p.m. And if the case seems exhausted, fresh *grape* juice or bottled grape juice, the unpasteurized kind, can be given, or *apple* juice, fresh or bottled, can be given. Average dose of juice for a cocker-size dog would be two tablespoons, morning and night.

Distemper Complications. If the disease is treated in its early stages there will be no complications. Beyond the slight disability of a cough, discharging eyes and nose, bouts of diarrhoea, and some fever, the dog will keep well, and the disease will generally have run its course, and the case be cured, within three weeks.

In fact, it should be a general rule that any sign of 'off colour' in the dog, i.e. listlessness, lack of appetite, abnormal sleepiness, or shivering, should be treated immediately by fasting and generous use of herbal antiseptic herbs, isolation from other dogs, and the taking of the case's temperature morning and night. If these precautions are always taken—and I have always taken them for my own dogs, goats, etc.—there will be no distemper disease as we know it today, and certainly there would be no complications.

But if first symptoms have been neglected, or the case is very in-bred from weak stock, or has been vaccinated recently, then any of the following complications could occur, and some of them are severe and dangerous to life. These distemper complications are: nervous disorders, including chorea; fits; paralysis; meningitis; chronic diarrhoea; jaundice; pneumonia and pleurisy; bronchitis; deranged heart; ulcers of eyes and mouth; eye keratitis; and more. (See treatments for all these ailments, as given in this chapter, in alphabetical order.)

Ailments and Their Treatments

Breeders' Reports on Distemper Cure

On account of the many new herbal treatments added to this new edition of my canine herbal, I now have space for only four reports, instead of the forty reports published in the first English edition, but I think they will lead many dog owners to utilize my herbal work; for, as declared Mrs. Joan Peck, of the famous Sakkara salukis (whose salukis were cured of hard pad by herbal treatment): 'I have heard of many people being converted from the orthodox to the herbal treatments, but I have yet to hear of a single case of the opposite conversion.'

Report No. 1.—Mrs. Joyce K. Gold (K. J. Fryer), Oxshott Cockers, Rabley Heath, Welwyn, breeder of many of England's greatest cockers, and a famous judge. 'For two years in succession I proved the complete success of your wonderful distemper treatment. Whereas in earlier years, puppies fed according to orthodox treatment when showing high temperature, invariably had complications and generally died. Following your treatment all my dogs made speedy recoveries and there have been no losses. . . . I have told so many people what a safe distemper method this is, and incidentally have cured many different dogs by phone that way. I shall always bless the day ten years ago when I got in touch with you, for the peace of mind your treatment of canine disorders has given me. I fear no illness now, as a few days' garlic treatment and fasting soon puts things right, but I must say my dogs keep *very* fit and free from ills, and it is many years since we have had anything serious to contend with.'

Report No. 2.—The Duchess of Laurino, Fenterwanson Pekinese, St. Teath, Cornwall, a Pekinese authority. 'I had twenty-seven Pekinese down with distemper, and treated them word for word as per your internal cleansing method. I lost one adult only. He started fits on the sixth day, but would have died whatever treatment he had been given, never having been normal. I had one young bitch which I despaired of saving. Her temperature continued for fourteen days. She was so weak that she could scarcely move, though in no way paralysed. Both eyes were badly ulcerated. Both lips and the nose sloughed off, leaving horrible pus on the open wounds. During all this time she had nothing beyond garlic and water. On the fifteenth morning I was rewarded by a wag of her tail. Next day she growled when I took her temperature; this

119

Ailments and Their Treatments

was down to normal and remained there. I continued the fast a further five days, then commenced the milk-honey diet, and in one week she was out and about again, with no trace of weakness. The bare places around her eyes and mouth remained, of course, for some time, but in every other way she was a perfectly normal dog. She has since been shown several times, winning first prizes at championship shows.

'The thing that impressed me most was that having shaken off the disease, even after prolonged fasts, there was no period of convalescence; they all seemed better in health than ever before. One dog contracted the disease despite the fact that he had been inoculated. Seven dogs who had never had it (given garlic), although in contact with the sick dogs, remained immune.

'One bitch only has been left with any disfigurement, this bitch continued running a slight temperature although apparently normal in every other way; unfortunately food was given, with the result that the temperature rose again and a second stage of the illness was entered upon with the tragic ending of an eye swollen almost entirely out of the socket and almost complete blindness in the other.

'Before trying your natural method I have nursed dogs of various breeds with distemper, *only one of which I saved*. These I nursed by giving strong beef tea or chicken broth at two-hourly intervals, pouring it down their mouths when refused, also giving them beaten raw eggs in milk and occasionally brandy. The result seemed to be that the dogs' stomachs were always working overtime, also their bowels, and—as I have said before—they invariably died most painful deaths.

'I find your treatment is a boon, as it is no trouble at all to carry out, and I am firmly convinced that if followed carefully and the dogs are kept clean and in warm, airy kennels, *all the dread of distemper can be forgotten*.'

Report No. 3.—Mrs. Betty Butterworth, Rodworth Gundog and Cocker Kennels, Thonon-les-Bains, Haute-Savoie, France (now: Butterworth, 246 E. 53, New York City 10022, N.Y., U.S.A.). Formerly Mme Coigny, Betty Butterworth was known throughout the French-speaking world, including North Africa, for her superb gundogs, which she exported all over the world. 'When as Madame Coigny I ran the "Of Rodworth" Cocker Spaniels, in Thonon, France, I started these kennels on orthodox lines, with cooked

Ailments and Their Treatments

foods, drugs, and vaccines, and changed to Natural Rearing after three miserable years of endless work, dying dogs and worried perpetually by enormous bills for veterinary surgeons and chemists. I changed to Natural Rearing after a bad outbreak of hard pad in which I lost fourteen animals. The change was not easy, my faith not very strong, and the constant desire to return to the old method of drugs and inoculations was with me for many months. However, I persisted, as you know, and the results were beyond anything I had hoped.

'During the next four years, with a basic stock of never less than twenty-five adults and rising at times to eighty dogs in the kennel, I lost only two animals and those through accidents and not illness. During these years, using only your method, I cured a newly purchased English bitch of Hard Pad. She was never isolated from the other stock and was the only case. Bored (if such a thing is possible) with the never-ending good health of my own stock and still not quite persuaded that the lack of illness was due to the treatment and feeding and not to my good luck, I began to search for sick dogs from other kennels and had among other cures great success in curing a bitch with bad chorea of the head and front legs, by fasting and then raw meat, seaweed powder, etc. She is now winning C.A.C.s in France for her owner and has bred some good stock.

'We went through a local epidemic of Hard Pad which destroyed many dogs in Thonon-les-Bains, without one case in the kennels. And this, in spite of the fact that many of the farmers and sportsmen, having heard of the methods used in the kennels, would arrive with their dogs, bringing them on to the premises in all stages of the disease.

'I think perhaps you realized my faith in Natural Rearing and my complete absence of fear when you brought your travel companion, Afghan hound, to me from Tunisia, with that strange skin infection from Arab desert dogs that we had neither of us seen before and which you so quickly cured with herbs gathered on our walks. It did not cross my mind to isolate your dog, or that any of mine would catch the complaint—none did, as you know. I had then and have now complete and utter faith in Natural Rearing, providing it is carried out thoroughly with no backsliding to drugs—plenty of free running exercise and good raw meat and strict attention paid to the usual kennel details of grooming and

Ailments and Their Treatments

cleanliness. I attribute much of my success in the show ring to the health of the dogs, and I made champions of many of them, including Ch. Doebank Dominant of Rodworth, Ch. Walener of Ware, Ch. Silver Teal of Rodworth, Ch. Melforts Colleen's Joy. The black bitch that you admired, Rhapsody of Rodworth, is now owned by Baron de Boc and needs only her working certificate to become an International champion; and the blue roan puppy Rodworth His Majesty of Hearts, which you picked out, is already an American champion.

'I hope one day to work again with animals and to enlarge my Natural Rearing experience with Farm Stock, but whilst I have had many opportunities to work along orthodox lines I confess I have not the courage to face again the disappointment, misery and death that are forever linked in my mind with the giving of drugs and inoculations.'

Report No. 4.—Viscountess Chelmsford, Beagles, etc., East Grinstead, Sussex. Famed as a judge of beagles, Viscount Chelmsford is one of the leading officials of the English Kennel Club. 'By following your treatment, honey and water, fasting and using garlic, a litter of Beagles, seriously ill, made a wonderful recovery from distemper; also one Cocker bitch, which had been suffering from skin trouble for two years, made a rapid recovery. The treatment has given every satisfaction and I am getting fine results. A Samoyed puppy had been digesting nothing before having the slippery-elm powder, as prescribed; now all is perfectly digested, and she is making excellent progress.' (Later, Crufts 1953: 'Since using your herbal treatments in the early nineteen-thirties, I have had much time in which to fully test all that you advise. I am more convinced than ever before, and follow strictly the advice in all your books.')

DROPSY. This condition of abnormal accumulation of fluid in the body is a serious ailment when found in the dog or cat. However, herbal treatment has achieved numerous cures of dropsy, mainly because there are many herbs which are curative. These are: *ground (dwarf) elder, dandelion, rosemary, parsley* seed, *yerba mansa (Mexican), couch grass.* The dog or cat should be fasted, given antiseptic herbal tablets and charcoal tablets. Follow the internal cleansing treatment carefully, but keep the case on a diet of fish (see Fish, page 31), in place of the raw meat, when full N.R.

Ailments and Their Treatments

diet is resumed. Give internally quantities of any of the above-listed curative herbs.

DYSENTERY. This is a very severe form of diarrhoea, which, if not treated properly and patiently, can have fatal results. There is often faulty temperature, either fever or subnormal temperature. Bowel discharge is very copious, very fluid, often orange in colour and foamy, with bad odour.

Treatment. Treat as for diarrhoea. Give *chamomile* tea, standard infusion, throughout; two tablespoons morning, midday, and night, average-size dog. *Apple* juice, a tablespoon morning and night, should also be given. A good Spanish remedy for dysentery, which I have seen used in severe typhus disease, is *rice* water. This is both soothing and only mildly astringent without being binding. Take six tablespoons (level) of rice grains, one and one-half pints of cold water. Bring to slow boil for two hours, keeping pan covered; remove from heat, and when tepid add two teaspoons honey and one-half teaspoon powdered *cinnamon*. Give a small cup thrice daily, give by spoon if necessary.

EARS: FOREIGN BODIES and WEAK MUSCLES. (For Ear Canker, see Canker.)

Foreign Bodies. Often dogs, hunting around in country places, get thorny material or sharp grass spines in ears. Dissolve by dropping into the ear a saltspoon of oil in which rue or rosemary has been infused. Later dry out the ear with cotton swabs soaked in buttermilk or very diluted witch hazel. Continue twice daily until cured.

Weak Muscles. This condition is not really an ailment: it is more a question of show merit as to whether or not the ears of special prick-eared breeds stand upright or remain drop-eared. But as herbs can help in restoring muscular tone, I have included this treatment.

Treatment. First, put the dog strictly on raw foods N.R. diet, including uncooked (raw) *maize* flour in the cereal feed. This will stimulate general muscular development. Externally, using standard infusion, make a lotion of *ivy* leaves, but of double strength, i.e. two handfuls of ivy to approximately one-half pint of water. Use the brew cold, massaging a small amount of it, twice daily, around the ear bases. Do not resort to taping or other artificial methods: rely on herbs and massage.

ECZEMA. This is often Nature's method of ridding the body,

Ailments and Their Treatments

especially the blood-stream, of accumulated toxins which have collected in the body from unnatural diet and/or lack of exercise. Also dirty, unbathed bodies are a cause. Streptococcal bacteria are often found in eczema pus, causing confusion with that disease. 'Strep' happens to be common bacteria found frequently where there is pus.

Treatment. An infusion of *nettle* plant, or *meadowsweet* flowers, internally, with also herbal antiseptic tablets. In severe eczema a short course of internal cleansing may be necessary. Externally, apply a brew of bramble or elder leaves and flowers, or a mixture of both. Some can be given internally also.

EYE AILMENTS. (See Cataract, etc.)

FITS. There are several forms of dog fits, caused by indigestion, or a distemper complication, or worms, or epilepsy. There are also the teething fits of puppyhood.

Treatment. Internal cleansing, with much use of honey. Give also *grape* juice, and black molasses. Herbs effective in curing fits are *wood sage*, *poppy* heads, *skullcap*, *rue*, and *rosemary*. Add minced raw *lettuce* and garden *mint* to the food, a heaped dessertspoon. For worm fits, see Worms. For epileptic, give strong doses of skullcap. An effective French peasant remedy is six *mistletoe* berries twice daily, before feeds.

Mrs. G. Petter (of the firm of Petter Oil Engines, Yeovil, Somerset) sent me a dramatic report concerning fits cure: 'I had taken my pet poodle to the veterinary surgery for destruction as his fits had been diagnosed as incurable. Returning from there I met Margaret Hemery,[1] breeder of Mayerling Boxers and Alsatians, who told me she had cured an Alsatian of "brain" distemper by following your treatment, and to get back the poodle if it had not already been put to sleep. The dog was still alive. Mrs. Hemery helped me and I carefully followed your treatment. The dog completely recovered and became very strong and normal.'

Cures of fits with herbs have been numerous. Chances of recovery are greater when dogs have not been given any serum shots previously, or have had suppression with 'quietener' drugs.

FLEAS, LICE, TICKS, AND OTHER SKIN VERMIN. These skin

---

[1] Margaret Hemery now lives at Santa Inez, California. She is well known in America as a judge of boxers and author of the book *Boxers* (Ernest Benn).

Ailments and Their Treatments

parasites are all blood-sucking and all do immense harm to the dogs which harbour them, especially to young stock; all dogs should be searched daily. The skin irritation caused by their presence keeps the dog in a constant state of unease; while the flea itself is known to be a carrier of a small species of tapeworm (*Dypylidum canicum*); the louse is suspect as a carrier—it is proved as a conveyor of typhus to humans—through its bite. Ticks can cause fevers in dogs, which can prove fatal.

Treatment. The first essential is to groom the dog and remove all loose hair, mats, scurf, etc. Then bathe thoroughly in a foamy bath of soap flakes, scrub well, also with a brush and using a bar of soap, preferably with olive oil. Do not forget to wash well the ears and tail. For perfect cleanliness, a second bathing with a good shampoo is advisable. When the dog is fully dry, dust over the entire body with a herbal insecticide, not forgetting inner ear flaps and under the tail. Avoid all chemicals, including DDT:[1] they are apt to do more damage to general health than the insects against which they are being used. A herbal rub for use when searching for vermin on the dog; moisten a pad of cotton wool or a piece of cotton cloth and sprinkle with a few drops each of oil of eucalyptus and spirit of camphor. This makes fleas easy to catch, and loosens lice and ticks.

Lemon lotion. Save all used *lemon* halves and place them in a gallon container, at least twenty-four halves to one gallon. Place the jar or container in the hot sunlight or pour hot water over the lemon. Let the lemon remain permanently in the water until pieces begin to turn mouldy, then remove and replace with fresh ones, squeezing hard the old ones into the water. Do not throw away any of the old lemon water which then remains. Rub the lemon lotion well into all parts of the dog's body to expel skin vermin. A little may be dropped into the ears. For a stronger lotion, add the juice from two lemons to every quart. (Keep the jar covered with a paper top—not greased paper.)

It must be stressed that it is useless to cleanse the dog's body of vermin while leaving his kennel untreated, for where there are but a few specks of dust a flea can remain and breed: and fleas, like most vermin, are extremely prolific. It is essential to the health of

[1] Now suppressed by law in many American states and Scandinavian countries, due to health hazards.

Ailments and Their Treatments

a dog that the kennel in which it lives should be lime-washed and
rested frequently, also the kennel runs, which should be dug over
and limed before being rested from use. No kennel or run ought
to be occupied for longer than a six-months' stretch without a
period of at least one month's resting. Wooden buildings and
earth (or even concrete) runs provide a harbouring place not only
for the external vermin, such as fleas and lice, but also for the eggs
of worms and for disease-provoking bacteria, which can remain
alive for years in the ground, according to the findings of Professor
Antoine Béchamp. Let it be known that real infestation by skin
vermin is not found where there are ideal kennel and rearing
conditions. A dog groomed daily and possessing a tough skin—a
natural accompaniment of true health—cannot harbour or prove
fit prey for many skin vermin. Cleanliness of animal and building
is the surest safeguard against vermin of all kinds, including rats,
mice, and cockroaches.

Where there has been severe vermin infestation in kennels, there
should be fumigation with either a sulphur candle or *cayenne
pepper*. For either method, do as follows: First seal all doors,
windows, wood cracks, etc. Then light the sulphur candle and well
seal up the outer door also. If cayenne pepper is used, a paraffin
stove should be placed in kennel or building, and lit, then on it
place an empty tin. Pour into this one ounce or so of cayenne, and
leave this to smoke slowly, sealing up the outer door also after
exit. Allow the pepper to burn and smoke overnight in a completely sealed building. After fumigation with either sulphur or
cayenne pepper, the place should be well ventilated for at least
twenty-four hours before dogs are allowed to enter it.

The advantage of the old-fashioned wooden-tub kennel or old
packing case was that, being cheap, it could easily be replaced by
a clean, new one, burning up the old and all worm ova and insect
vermin along with it! Expensive kennel buildings are a mistake.
Better to have many cheap ones which can be rested and/or replaced sometimes.

In warm weather all bedding should be removed. Clean sacks
can be given if desired.

A herbal insecticide lotion. During wet weather it is not possible
to use a dry, powdered insecticide. Here is a home-made lotion of
proved effective action and entirely beneficial to canine health.
Pour one-half pound herbal insecticide powder, such as my own

Ailments and Their Treatments

formula—five-herbs powder—or powdered *derris* root or *tobacco* dust, into a glass flask big enough to hold two quarts (the big bottles sold with spring or purified water are suitable). Next, add two ounces of oil of *eucalyptus* and one quart of pure alcohol (or beer can be used with excellent results). Cork tightly to prevent the escape of the natural herbal oils released by the alcohol. Set this to steep for four days. Shake the contents well, morning and night. The lotion must now be filtered to prevent over-fermentation. Do this through a large funnel packed with cheesecloth or cotton. Have ready another large bottle capable of holding at least two gallons, or have two bottles capable of holding one gallon each. The alcohol lotion can now be diluted to a quantity of two gallons and yet retain pungency sufficient to destroy skin parasites. If there is any fermentation later on, it does not matter, it will increase the pungency of the lotion, and it is for external use, not internal.

If the odour of eucalyptus oil is objected to for house pets, then the more expensive oil of *rosemary* can be used, the same two-ounce amount. Good herbal stores stock this or can obtain it on order. For use, rub the lotion well into the skin over the entire animal, but keep from close contact with the eyes.

GASTRITIS. This is always caused through either faulty diet or worm infestation; in the former cause the trouble is especially due to the long-term feeding of cooked foods and to the giving of irritant appetite-stimulating drugs in 'condition'-powder form.

Treatment. (See Diarrhoea.) An infusion of *parsley* leaves is also recommended. A long fast is often necessary. When the fast has been ended, use should be made of steamed parsley roots, well minced and fed with the cereal. (No salt is to be added during the steaming—which should be carried out in the smallest possible amount of water, that water being retained and mixed in with the cereal—a dog can obtain all the salt necessary to health through the medium of the seaweed powder, as given in the N.R. diet.) In orthodox treatment it is usual to limit drinking-water strictly. I break this rule and give as much fluid as desired, only I add half of *chamomile*.

HARD PAD AND BRAIN DISTEMPER (CANINE ENCEPHALITIS). The disease is usually classed as a virus ailment and, like distemper, its real cause has not been proved. I link the disease very closely with canine distemper, and I further believe from careful

127

Ailments and Their Treatments

observation that it is an actual form of distemper. It can be cured by the same method, though it is usually held to be nearly incurable by those who treat the disease by orthodox methods. I consider the disease curable, though not so easily as distemper, for animals which produce hard-pad disease symptoms have reached a very substandard state of health, and their bodies will require very careful and prolonged internal cleansing and dieting in order to attain normal health. It is far more prevalent in Europe than in the Americas. Common symptoms are: diarrhoea, which is seldom absent as an early symptom of canine encephalitis; also an excessively moist nose, usually with drops of water continually appearing there; similar moisture is frequently found around the eyes, although there is no yellow mucus discharge, or from the nostrils, typical of common distemper. There is always a raised temperature, for there cannot be inflammation of the nerves without any indication of fever, and it is the general body nerves which are first inflamed—one of the causes of diarrhoea, for diarrhoea can well be produced by purely nervous irritation of the intestinal tract, and therefore nothing at all is gained by merely checking the diarrhoea flow and leaving the nerves still sick and irritated. There is always a staring coat, and usually the inner ear flaps are very hot, and some discharge is also seen there. It is always much later, and sometimes not at all, that the foot pads—and in some cases the nostril pads—thicken and become leathery, and finally harden and become almost without feeling, in the same way as skin areas do after long-lasting follicular mange—only in hard pad it is more exaggerated. With this stage are found the brain symptoms, shown by the staggering gait of the affected animal and constant whimpering which cannot be suppressed by command, the dog acting involuntarily, and described as 'insane'; until in the last stages it is a raving madness similar to pure meningitis.

Internal Treatment. Similar to canine distemper, although more intensive, for hard pad is indeed dangerous, whereas distemper is a simple disease to treat. Once the typical symptoms have been verified—diarrhoea, very wet nose (and possibly eyes), fever (usually a temperature of an unvarying 103° F.)—the only possible treatment to prevent death is a complete fast on honey and water only. (Try to obtain pure honey, not the syrupy, often pasteurized substitute for the pure thing.) Medicine should be: a daily dose of antiseptic herbs, especially *garlic* and *rue*, double the dose as pre-

128

Ailments and Their Treatments

scribed for canine distemper, given each morning. Follow this with a twice-daily dose of a brew made from *potato* peelings, made as follows: shred a small cupful of potato peelings; pour over this three cupfuls of cold water; bring to boil and simmer for about ten to fifteen minutes, until the water turns to a light brown. Allow the peelings to stand and steep off the fire for at least two hours, then squeeze out the juice. Dosage is two tablespoons twice daily for big breeds; one tablespoon twice daily, medium breeds; two teaspoons, small breeds. Give also a large dose of vegetable tablets, made to my formula, and being pure chlorophyll extracted from nettles and meadow grasses and *comfrey*. A laxative is necessary during fasting—see Internal Cleansing Chart, page 99. This appears to be a large amount of dosing, but the disease is a serious one; and it is far preferable to have such work in the early stage of the disease, and cure resulting, than the enormous amount of work entailed in caring for a case of brain fever, which state, when allied to hard pads and nostrils, becomes very serious indeed.

If there are definite brain-disorder symptoms, *skullcap* treatment should replace the potato brew internally until the nerves are soothed and normalized.

Hard pad taken before brain-disorder sets in is curable. I have achieved many cures with the fasting-herbs-potato treatment. (Potato-skins' brew has a remarkable effect upon diseased tissue, and combined with garlic, on my prescribing, has even cured the considered-to-be-incurable fistulous withers of horses. This treatment, being given much publicity in agricultural journals in England, aroused wide interest and helped to achieve my B.B.C. radio talk on many kinds of animals which I have saved with herbs.) Peasant farmers in Ireland use potato skins for sick animals and, incidentally, were using bread mould (penicillin) dissolved in water—as animal medicine and also for their own ailments—long before English scientists ever 'discovered' the medicinal value of the mould fungi group.

It is interesting to note that in an old herbal book of the Mexican army, a brew of potato peelings, used externally, is given as a cure for the dread typhus fever.

External Treatment. Make poultice boots from a piece of cotton, linen, or sacking—nothing woollen—spread with a plaster of pulped, boiled potato peelings, or oatmeal or barley flour. The boots must be kept in place with adhesive tape or some strong tape. Change the boots every day, allowing half a day *without* boots before each new application. The boots must be very loose-fitting around the pads, but tied firmly up the leg.

Warning. The cessation of the diarrhoea is no sign of a full cure; normal temperature, maintained steadily for three days, is the most favourable sign of cure, and permits milk and, later, other foods, to be added to the honey-water diet. Continue to take the temperature daily; in case of relapse, continue for at least eighteen days in all hard-pad cases.

A further warning is against the use of any drugs of the sulphonamide group. The indiscriminate use of these *highly dangerous* drugs is quite possibly one cause of this disease, allied with the presence of toxins of the distemper type. It is notable that in cows —animals which react very badly to chemical medicine—sulphonamide treatment is frequently followed by disease of the hoofs. There may well be some link between the modern popularity of these dangerous drugs and the corresponding frequency of hard pad and brain distemper, for mental disorders are another common after-effect of the sulphonamides.

Prevention of hard pad. As I have already stated, Natural Rearing is a sure preventive. When dogs are known to have been exposed to infection, disinfect their blood-stream with Nature's most potent disinfectant—herbs, especially *garlic* and *rue*. Be unfailing in this habit.

Finally, I want to bring attention once more to the prevalent error of classifying all sorts of minor canine disorders as being hard pad, now that this disease has 'leapt into popularity', taking the interest from the once equally important streptococcal infection disease. Mr. Leo Wilson, F.Z.S., writes sensibly on this matter: 'In assessing these cases [hard pad], however, one must always be sure that diagnosis has been correct. When a "new" disease becomes an epidemic the label is applied loosely to a variety of cases which may not be the disease at all and consequently the cures effected do not help in the fight against the major foe.'

The spreading of superstitious fears concerning diseases of humans and animals is often the work of serum 'merchants' preliminary to their marketing of a new serum.

I am grateful to Miss May Rodgers for her detailed report on her success with hard-pad treatment, which I give herewith. Miss Rodgers writes with authority, having cured the disease on three

Ailments and Their Treatments

occasions. Mr. Leo Wilson introduces her work as follows, in a paragraph headed 'Hard Pad Cures' in his London Wire (*Our Dogs*): 'More than one of my readers mentions the use of garlic in one form or another, both as a cure and preventative. One writer, Miss M. Rodgers, of Leeds, is particularly warm in her praise of garlic, which she used in conjunction with starvation treatment. She claims successes against Hard Pad with this method as long as twelve years ago.

' "Miss May Rodgers, Gledhow Chows, 66 Upland Grove, Leeds, Yorkshire.

' "I first had this disease in my kennels about twelve years ago, and treated the dogs as for distemper. I wrote to Juliette de Baïracli-Levy (when she had distemper kennels in London, at Talbot Road, Bayswater) and she wrote back that she had never come across the disease where the pads hardened, but would like to know the detailed symptoms, and what progress I made, etc. I kept her fully informed, and she said she thought that, seeing one particular dog was ravenously hungry *and* running a temperature, his brain *must* be affected (which proved to be). I eventually got him better, but he was always nervous. His litter brother (my blue stud Chin-Cha—retired from stud now) would not have *any* food, not even honey or milk, and he had no after-effects.

' "Since this experience I have had Hard Pad twice in my kennels, the last time four years ago, when I again wrote J. de Baïracli-Levy, and she suggested that I poultice the feet. Though I do not poultice any more, my experience having found foot coverings to be unsatisfactory.

' "As to *treatment*: (I have not so far lost *one* dog or bitch.) I starve the same as for distemper (internal cleansing), and give garlic night and morning—one tablet per dose. I do not touch the dog's pads except to rinse them with aired boiled water once or twice, *until* the dog starts to tear them off himself, then I leave them *severely* alone. Rinse the mouth and clean the teeth with lemon and water (one and a half teaspoonfuls of pure lemon juice to two tablespoonfuls of water) and do not 'fuss' the dog, simply keep him quiet and warm (not in a hot room, he does better in his own kennel). I have found that the cases want plenty of water and also that the temperature is often *below* normal at commencement, though it rises as the dog's feet harden. When the foot pads are coming off, I put my dogs on the milk or milk-and-water diet, with

131

addition of a teaspoonful of honey. The slippery elm, etc., powder form, is good to use before the dogs are returned to normal diet, especially useful to check the tendency to bowel looseness which is also one of the true early symptoms of Hard Pad disease (the only other commencing symptom that I have observed is the dog's habit of walking very *carefully*, as if he had a touch of rheumatism in his front legs. There are no other symptoms at commencement).

' "I hope that my experience with Hard Pad will be of use to other dog owners. I shall be very pleased if I can help to cure this disease and encourage other people to try this simple treatment."'

Mrs. Gisela Meyer-Frank, Karl-Muller-Str., 8, Dusseldorf, Germany, tells me how herbal method is becoming accepted in her country. She cured her own Afghan of a severe attack of hard pad, using my herbal treatment under supervision of her veterinary surgeon who was 'very interested in your method. We read together some brand-new veterinary books and I found the same as you told me: garlic, green herbs, raw food, eucalyptus, and watercress, against Hard Pad'.

HEART WEAKNESS AND DISEASE. The treatment of all the many types of heart weakness and disease is similar. In the main, the heart should be relieved of all unnecessary work, through diet reform to reduce superfluous flesh and free the blood-stream of toxic accumulations which are so damaging to the heart and the blood-stream in general—for the health of the heart is largely governed by the state of health of the entire blood system of the organism. Exercise should not be curtailed. Active exercise is necessary for complete food digestion; otherwise, the blood-stream becomes impure and the heart is further harmed.

Treatment. The specific remedies for heart disorders are: rosemary and honey. An infusion of *rosemary* should be used, one level teaspoon of pure honey being added to every tablespoon of the rosemary infusion. Rosemary herb has all of the three medicinal properties necessary in heart treatment: it is tonic, cleansing, and also a nervine. Honey is the only known heart stimulant and restorant which is not a drug and which is not habit forming. Dandelion leaves and watercress should be given daily on the meat feed, for their rich iron content, and the potassium and copper content of dandelion which has an important effect on heart restoration. Regular fasting and use of mild laxatives, such as rhubarb root or senna, should also play an important part in all heart treatments.

Avoid digitalis, the popular heart medicine; from the simple herb foxglove the chemists have made a dangerous medicine. Flowers of lily of the valley are a very good heart tonic, but expensive. Heartsease (wild pansy) is good.

HEPATITIS (*Liver Disease*). This disease has a short incubation period and can develop and be passed on to another dog within three days or so. There is often some pus in the eyes, bad breath, great lassitude, rapid wasting, irregular bowel action. This is one more hitherto-rare disease now considered as common. That it is so severe and so general, and attacks an organ greatly influenced by diet, is one more proof of the terrible harm done to dogs by unnatural diet.

Treatment. Isolate the case owing to its contagion. Treat as for jaundice (see Jaundice). Keep the case quiet and warm, as temperature often drops below normal.

HIP-DYSPLASIA. This abnormality is shown by a stumbling gait. Faulty diet, deficient in natural bone-forming foods, and lack of hard exercise, are the basic causes.

Treatment. There is none, other than prevention in puppyhood by following Natural Rearing. Give bone-forming cereals, especially oats. Also give the herb comfrey, which has such a beneficial effect on bone-formation; its old country name is knit-bone. Dogs also need full access to sunlight.

HYSTERIA. The causes are many, the disease certainly not being caused by any specific bacteria, although many canine writers still claim that that is so. The many causes can readily be summed up in the two words which occur with such frequency in this book—incorrect rearing. Three contributory causes are: the presence of worms in large numbers, hereditary nerve weakness, and —boredom. The third cause, that of boredom, deserves further comment. The unnatural imprisoning of dogs in kennels for long intervals, or in small runs, without the provision of sufficient daily outside exercising, leads to a form of either mental depression or unnatural excitability in dogs so treated, a dog's nature being such that it is supplied with very highly developed feelings of affection and also the faculty to take a keen and intelligent interest in the life of its own home—or kennel. Therefore, as is often the case, the dogs are cut off from all outside interests, and the kennel owners have little time to spend in the company of the dogs, which are kept more as mere breeding machines than living creatures. It is understandable that the dogs so treated should become fretful and also ultra-sensitive to the slightest degree of excitement, and therefore prone to develop attacks of nervous hysteria at the most trifling cause. If this hysteria is to be prevented, it will therefore be seen that two reforms in the common life of the kennel dog are necessary; correct feeding, in order to ensure strong nerves as well as at the same time prevent worm infestation, and the provision for the dog of a way of life in which it can fulfil those special purposes for which it was created; namely, that of being friend, companion, and guard to man, worker—shepherd and hunter— and also destroyer of harmful rodent vermin and serpents. Then, above all, supply ample, active exercise.

Treatment. When a dog develops attacks of hysteria, the most important contribution towards successful cure is rest in a darkened room, combined with fasting, the full internal cleansing treatment then being followed, with a return to a fluid diet whenever further attacks of the hysteria occur. The same herbal treatment as for fits should be followed. I must also mention the fact that because hysteria is such a noisy and generally alarming ailment, breeders are frequently over-anxious to keep the dog artificially quiet by drugging; the commonest medicines used for drugging being bromide and luminol. These two drugs have been wittily and truly described by a medical writer as being 'those super Shylocks which demand a thousand per cent interest for any temporary relief they give'. How true indeed that statement is! The prolonged use of bromides (and other 'doping' drugs of that class) develops a peculiar state in the body. There is the case of the bromide drugs (the medical term for that state is bromism), a few symptoms of which state are herewith given: dilated pupils; development of acne on various parts of the body, especially the head and face; a fetid, bromine breath; slow and feeble action of the heart; breathlessness; cold extremities; various mental conditions, such as weakness and confusion of mind, and a type of general intoxication.

The one medicine that can be safely given in hysteria is the *skullcap* infusion: that herb is no suppressive drug, it actually feeds and builds the nerves as well as soothing them. *Rosemary, rue, hops, lime blossom* are also good. The one food which has a

Ailments and Their Treatments

curative effect in hysteria is honey. *Rose*-hip syrup and *black-currant* syrup are beneficial.

INGROWING EYELIDS. This is often hereditary and can be cured only by surgical operation. I have found the trouble frequent among wire, smooth, and Airedale terriers, and many breeds of toy dogs, especially poodles. The operation is simple and inexpensive. Bathe the sore eyes with *rosemary* infusion, this being antiseptic and healing. The following herbs all make good eye lotions: *balm*, *chickweed*, *dock*, *quince* seeds, *poppyseed* heads. Diet can also greatly improve eye health. *Linseed* soup, grated raw *carrot*, cooked *carrot*, *watercress* and all whole-grain cereals.

INTERDIGITAL CYSTS. (See Abscess.)

JAUNDICE. This ailment is commonly called the 'yellows', named for the yellow hue that dyes the entire body surface, even the gums and eyeballs. The causes of jaundice are many, and include: congestion of the liver—frequently brought about as a sequela of distemper, or through a severe chilling; blocking of the bile duct by the passing of a gallstone or the entrance of a round worm. There is also a form of contagious leptospiral jaundice said to be caused by rats, typical cases, however, of this having been found where no rats or mice could possibly have been responsible; serum injections are given for this jaundice. They are given with the admission of 'kill or cure'; they usually kill. There is also preventive inoculation, which itself is more deadly to young stock in its after-effects than are even distemper inoculations. The one unfailing jaundice preventive is sound rearing according to the laws of Nature.

Treatment. Infusion of *dandelion* leaves and root, the two infusions to be given mixed together in equal parts; for preparation of the root, see preparation of couch grass (under Bladder Troubles), also *toad-flax* or blue pimpernel in infusion. An infusion of *rhubarb* stems is also very effective: two ounces of stem to one half pint of water cooked into a thick syrup, with honey added. And *pomegranate* juice when in season, an average dose being two dessertspoons morning and night. Externally, a paste of common *mustard* can be made into a poultice and applied hot to the region of the liver. A course of internal cleansing, with garlic dosing, must be followed; but when the milk-honey stage is reached, the milk should be given sour and skimmed, and only half the usual quantity of honey given—both measures being in-

135

tended to relieve the work of the liver, which is the organ of the body most concerned in fats and sugar digestion and storage.

Extraordinarily good results have been obtained in the treatment of jaundice by the above method, despite the fact that jaundice is considered one of the most fatal of all canine ailments.

Note. I must repeat that the entire success of the jaundice treatment depends upon strict fasting long enough for the liver to have become cleansed, and the bile to have been cleared from the blood-stream and body tissues.

KERATITIS. This is a clouding over of the eyes; their natural opaqueness vanishes and they often turn an unsightly solid-looking blue.

Treatment. Give the dog a period of internal cleansing. Give as medicine: *carrot* juice, carrots—shredded raw and/or cooked, corn meal, *linseed* tea, to improve the health of the eyes through diet.

For eye-bathing lotion, see Cataract treatment.

KIDNEY TROUBLE, INFLAMMATION, ETC. (See Bladder Troubles for complete treatment.) An infusion of *parsley* leaves should replace the couch-grass infusion. The internal cleansing method has given outstanding results in kidney diseases; numerous incurables have been cured. Cleavers plant infused in cold milk is effective. Also parsnips, grated, raw; can be rolled into balls, with thick honey.

LEATHER-SKIN (OR ELEPHANT SKIN) DISEASE. The cause of this serious ailment may be abnormal secretions of the glands; in one form it is the pituitary gland, in another it is the sebaceous glands: sometimes a hormone deficiency. Origin is considered to be internal as with most skin ailments; even ringworm and mange are influenced by internal health. In leather-skin, the skin thickens like leather; if not checked and if the condition spreads unduly, there will be no recovery.

Treatment. Treat as a glandular disease (see Obesity). Give an abundance of *seaweed* and *garlic* internally; externally massage the skin with garlic infusion in castor oil (see preparation under Abscess).

LEPTOSPIROSIS (LEPTOSPIRA CANICOLA, LEPTOSPIRA ICTERO-HAEMORRHAGIAE). We can classify these two ailments as 'new'. Almost unheard of when I commenced veterinary work nearly thirty years ago, they are now so commonplace that dog owners,

Ailments and Their Treatments

especially in Europe, are being urged to have their dogs vaccinated with a triple vaccine, to protect not only against canine distemper and hard pad but also against these two forms of leptospirosis (and while going 'the whole hog' in vaccines, why not a fourth shot to protect against contagious hepatitis?). It is good to know that one of the world's most famous dogs, Ch. Shirkhan of Grandeur, of America, has never been vaccinated against anything, and yet he has travelled with his owner, following his great triumph of Best of All Breeds, at Westminster Show, New York, 1959, attending championship shows throughout the United States and winning Group after Group prizes, and has also travelled on invitation to Venezuela.

Healthy dogs do not get leptospiral infections; they, again, come to the ones reared by unnatural methods. Leptospira canicola is often called 'the lamp-post disease', as city dogs, especially males, are said to infect themselves from sniffing around urine-soaked lamp posts, on which infected dogs have urinated. The bacteria is corkscrew-shaped and infects the kidneys. Infected dogs become very emaciated, blood is often passed in the urine. As many as 50 per cent of dogs in most cities of the world are said to be infected. One should count N.R. dogs among the disease-free other 50 per cent because they will not get the infection. Healthy kidneys resulting from healthy feeding give them their immunity.

Symptoms of L. canicola are, refusal of food, vomiting, fetid breath, abdomen tender to the touch, blood sometimes passed in the strong-smelling urine, and a rapid loss of weight.

L. icterohaemorrhagiae is supposed to be rat-borne and affects the liver, causing internal bleeding and rapid death. A normally healthy liver will resist attack. I should also say that leptospiral ailments are often made scapegoats for common canine distemper. Cases which have been vaccinated against distemper cannot be admitted by the veterinary surgeon as having developed the disease, therefore it is called leptospirosis instead: little wonder that the percentage of town dogs suffering from this 'new' disease is now put as high as fifty dogs out of every hundred.

Treatment. Exactly as for canine distemper. Fasting and resting the case, giving antiseptic herbs, also honey. For the kidney infection, see also Bladder Troubles; for the liver infection, see Jaundice.

Although leptospiral jaundice is considered to be almost invariably fatal, many complete cures have been achieved, using simple herbal method.

LIMBS, FRACTURES OF. Fractures of limbs are quite frequent in the dog; it is usually the long bones of the leg which are injured; occasionally the ribs. There are three kinds of fracture: simple, when the bone is broken in one place only and there is no wound; compound, when there is a wound in addition to the fracture and communicating with the fracture; and comminuted, when the bone is smashed in several pieces.

Treatment. The simple fracture does not usually present much difficulty; it is with the two other forms that much care has to be used. The first thing to do is reduce the fracture—which means the setting of the broken bones in their natural position. The next thing is the splinting and the bandaging of the injured parts, securing the limb in such a way that the broken bone-ends are prevented from moving out of place once they have been set, keeping the bones in rightful position in order to ensure the uniting of the broken bone-ends: this process is always a difficult one owing to the dog's natural dislike of any coverings on any part of the body, especially on the legs. (It is known that when the wild deer sustain a broken leg, as the result usually of a fall from cliffside, or elsewhere, they keep the injured limb inactive and raised from the ground, until the breakage has healed. Such breakages, through falls, are not uncommon among the wild deer, whose dread of man as a result of the terrible hound-hunting persecution to which they are subjected, causes them to inhabit dangerous cliffsides and other similar places. But I have yet to see a wild deer with a crooked leg.) I think that it might often prove the best policy where a nervous dog is concerned, to allow the dog to heal its own limb, merely keeping the dog confined in some quiet place until the limb has healed sufficiently to allow the taking of active exercise again. Internally, give an infusion of *broom*, the tender shoots and the leaves of that shrub having remarkable power in promoting the uniting of the ends of fractured bones. Wild animals with broken limbs will seek out the broom bushes at such times.

Comfrey, a common wild herb, also cultivated as cattle fodder, is another important bone-healing herb. Indeed, a common name for comfrey is 'knit-bone'. Give this herb internally, chopped finely and mixed with the food, also as an infusion, standard method,

Ailments and Their Treatments

two tablespoons dose, morning and night. Then further use the infusion on cotton cloths, cold, thoroughly soaking the cloths and padding them around the broken limb: if a plaster setting is used, this is not possible. As the cloths dry, more brew should be added, to make a cold herbal pack. Comfrey encourages the speedy formation of new bone. A substance, *allantoin*, is largely responsible for comfrey's bone-knitting property.

Drinking raw goat's milk, in the experience of a famous goat breeder, Mrs. Lucy Tyler, Flemington, New Jersey, is a great aid in mending broken bones.

When I was in Texas, U.S.A., recently, I met Miss MacDonald White, of Associated Press, a follower of N.R. for years. She brought me a black and tan Afghan hound to see. The Afghan had fractured a foreleg some months before. I was asked to examine her legs, as the owner vowed I could never tell which one had been broken. She was correct, I could not tell, even when in movement. The Afghan had been treated by the herbal method that I am here describing.

But when the fracture is of such a nature that the bones must be kept in position by splinting, then the greatest care is required to make sure that the splinting does not interfere with the blood circulation; which interference would naturally prevent all healing and could produce a septic or even gangrenous condition. It is this very factor which makes me opposed to the modern veterinary method of tight setting in plaster of Paris, or other settings of that class. Such a setting might answer for a simple fracture, but in a compound or especially in a comminuted fracture, plaster of Paris settings are not to be recommended, and I have formed this opinion from bitter experience. I have seen the badly fractured leg of an exceptionally healthy hound puppy set in plaster, the hair having been clipped off the leg and the plaster applied to the skin without any padding of any sort to relieve pressure; the result of such unnatural treatment being that so much fluid and bad blood collected in the pinched limb that at length the swollen leg burst its way through the plaster; the condition of the limb then being such that destruction of the puppy was necessary. I most definitely prefer the old-fashioned method of splinting and lightly bandaging, for that method does at least allow the leg to breathe—and when the bandaging is lightly applied, does certainly permit normal circulation, which, of course, is essential to healing. There is a

139

gypsy method of setting broken limbs—which method is still in use on sheep farms in the West Country of England—and that is setting in 'containers' made from plant stems or tree branches. When a dog, sheep, or other animal fractures a limb, either a stout *cabbage* stump or *elder* branch is taken, and the pith removed from the centre, the stalk or branch then padded with some soft material (*sphagnum moss*, because of its antiseptic properties, would be excellent for this, or the healing *elder* leaves), and the stalk or branch then fixed round the fractured limb, and held in position by light bandaging. If the limb is a very broad one, then several stalks or branches can be placed edge to edge and then lightly bound in position. The advantages of this natural herbal splint are many: both stem and branch are porous and admit air to the limb; they are slightly pliant; their inner sides are soft and will not form hard ridges in the manner of plaster; but, above all, the herbal splints are themselves possessed with healing properties, and will therefore encourage Nature in her natural reparative work. For instance, the old herbalists used to prescribe cabbage water as a lotion for bathing bruised, swollen, aching, or gouty legs. The leaves of the *holly* tree, when trimmed of their prickles and bruised, and applied to fractured limbs in the area of the fracture, are claimed by the gypsies to have remarkable powers of uniting the bone ends so that they are left in as strong a condition as they ever were before the fracturing. Another important advantage of the herbal splints is that if the injured limb should swell it is only necessary to loosen the bandage and increase the space between the splint edges encircling the limbs; whereas, in plaster settings, it would be necessary to strip off the plaster altogether, for resetting, which procedure would certainly cause the animal much pain, and at the same time might well cause a further breakage of the injured bone ends.

The main points of natural treatment of fracture are, therefore: a natural setting of the limb, which means very light splinting and bandaging at first, during the time that the injured limb usually is swollen and tender (the splinting can always be tightened as the leg heals and the swelling disappears); the most careful daily inspection of the limb to make sure that the circulation is not being interfered with (not possible when plaster settings are being used); the provision of both quiet and rest, the dog not being permitted to take any active exercise at all for the first ten to fourteen days

Ailments and Their Treatments

following the fracture of the limb; and, further, a course of internal cleansing to help the body in its healing work; fasting and fluid diet, followed by only very light diet—of importance when no exercise is being taken.

When ribs are fractured, the area of the ribs should merely be wrapped around with a broad bandage placed so that the broken rib ends are kept in position but not made of a tightness to interfere with the animal's breathing. Rest and dieting are the other essentials. Bind bruised *holly* leaves, trimmed of prickles, over the rib area, beneath outer bandage, to increase healing.

LIVER AILMENTS. (See Jaundice and Hepatitis.)

MANGE. This is a severe parasitical disease which occurs in two forms, sarcoptic and follicular, the former being the more common of the two and the more contagious, but fortunately the more readily curable. As mange attacks also the fox and wolf, there is indication that it can be equally parasitical upon the quite healthy animal; therefore, keep stock away from other animals showing signs of mange skin disease.

The two kinds of mange parasites are small, louse-type mites, invisible to the naked eye. They bury beneath the skin and increase with great rapidity. Cases of follicular mange often look as if they have been sprayed all over with gunshot, so numerous are the skin eruptions. The skin further turns elephant grey, hair falls, and an unpleasant mousy smell becomes noticeable.

Sarcoptic mange is often confused with eczema and vice versa. But there are differences. Eczema means the formation of small mattery sores, spotty eruptions; while mange usually shows large wet patches and especially favours the back and back of the neck. There is also a falling out of the hair in mange, whereas in eczema the hair usually becomes matted with pus, but remains on the body. The presence of other skin vermin, especially lice, will also set up intense skin irritation which can be confused with mange or eczema; the smallness of the dog lice makes them difficult to detect.

Treatment. This, understandably, should be external principally, but in order to effect a complete cure, the state of the dog's general health should be improved also, for the tough, vital skin of the dog in sound health offers much resistance to the mange parasites: it is usually the skin of sickly animals that is attacked. Some animal experts go so far as to say that mange can be cured entirely

141

Ailments and Their Treatments

by corrective dieting and internal medicament. I consider that patient external treatment also is essential once the teeming parasites have established themselves in the skin tissues.

Complete fumigation of collars, leads, grooming equipment, kennels, and runs, is essential (see Fleas, etc.).

Herewith are four effective cures for both forms of mange. All are non-chemical and do not contain grease, which I consider to be very detrimental in the treatment of parasitical skin ailments, for it protects the tiny parasites and also they feed on it.

Bathe the dog thoroughly before applying any of these following treatments, using both soap flakes and a bar of olive-oil soap. Repeat the bath once each week throughout the treatment.

Herbal insecticide-alcohol lotion. (See treatment of fleas, lice, etc., this chapter, for recipe.) The lotion must be applied to every inch of the dog's body, not forgetting the very tail tip and around the toes; only avoid the eyes. Friction well into the skin.

Lemon-peel lotion. (For recipe, see under Treatment of Fleas, etc.) When *pomegranates* are available, their peel can be added to this lemon lotion with great advantage to the treatment. Use the skins from three pomegranates to every nine lemons.

In sunless localities the lemon skins must be treated with hot water and simmered for several minutes, keeping the pan covered. Then remove from the flame and allow to steep. Do not take the lemon peel out of the water throughout its use.

Garlic lotion. Follow the recipe for herbal insecticide in alcohol, as given under Fleas, but add finely minced *garlic*, six whole roots (meaning approximately forty small cloves), to the herbal powder, using the garlic in place of the oil of eucalyptus.

Violet and red clover lotion. Take a handful of each of these herbs; for the clover use both flowers and leaves. Pour over the herbs one quart of cold water, bring to a boil, and simmer for approximately three minutes. Keep covered throughout. Steep and use. Do not strain.

Garlic-elder lotion. Slice up three whole roots of *garlic*, consisting of about twenty cloves, and add to this two handfuls of finely cut *elder* leaves and stalks. Place all in a pan with one quart of cold water, bring to a boil, and simmer slowly for half an hour. Keep covered throughout. Remove from heat. Do not strain. Allow to brew for at least seven hours, still keeping covered. The lotion is then ready for use. Soak large pieces of cotton or towelling in the brew and friction the entire body very well. Two to three table-spoons of the brew can also be given internally early morning and at night.

For further internal treatment, if the case is very badly infected, a short fast may be necessary to clean the blood-stream. Give strong doses (double normal dose) of herbal antiseptic tablets.

Before closing this section mention should be made of con-stitutional hereditary mange, found especially in chows and dachs-hunds. Animals infected in this way should *never* be bred from. Unfortunately this rule is often ignored if a dog possesses good show points. Treatment for such mange is largely *internal*. Make much use of *seaweed*, giving a double dose, also herbal antiseptic tablets. Feed a strictly N.R. raw foods diet.

Here is an interesting and typical mange-cure testimonial. The photograph of the dog mentioned is shown in plate 23. From Mrs. Helen Balk-Roesch, Loerrach 2, Baden, Germany: 'I owe you a debt of gratitude in connection with your herbal canine book. I raised my small Scottish terrier according to your method. Friends of mine, the Gerhard Gunthers, also of Loerrach, brought me their year-old dog of the same breed. He was suffering from follicular mange and the attending veterinary had already decreed the killing of the little dog, as well as the complete disinfection of the apartment.

'I bought your herbal book of which I had heard. After ten months of constant and devoted care, I was able to return the dog to his owners, completely cured. Nobody would have believed it, but with use of garlic inside and out, the little dog recovered completely. The illness was incredible. Not one hair on his whole body, sores full of pus and with deep holes so that one could see almost to his bones in many places. It was a difficult task, but well worth it. Now little Bimbo has a beautiful black coat just like my own two Scottish terriers, which I bring up exactly to your diet chart. My Nature dogs differ markedly from other dogs, not only in their behaviour and intelligence, but also in the thickness of their beautiful coats.

'I wish to express my heartfelt thanks to you for this wonderful work you are doing for animals. The doctor who attended the sick dog originally was surprised no end when he saw the animal again after cure. He could hardly believe his eyes!'

MENINGITIS. (See Hard Pad.)

Ailments and Their Treatments

METRITIS. Metritis is a disease of the womb, which affects bitches of all ages, including maiden bitches, and is more common than is generally supposed; many bitches suffering from vaginal discharge are undiagnosed cases of metritis. The cause of metritis is usually held to be a germ which attacks the womb, but I have more faith in the less-known theory: that metritis is nothing more than a symptom of severe catarrh. The word 'catarrh' is derived from the Greek and means 'a flowing down'; and this flow of mucus can well occur in any part of the body where there are mucous membranes; we thus get colitis in the bowels, metritis in the womb, and so forth. The disease is distinguishable by an unpleasant-smelling discharge flowing from the vagina, the discharge being of a pinkish hue, and when very copious is usually accompanied by a rise of temperature.

Treatment. An infusion of *wild rose* fruits (or garden rose). When not available the leaves can be used, but they are far inferior to the fruits—the hips. The hips should be well crushed, and then brewed in the usual way. The infusion is improved by the addition of *witch-hazel* extract, one half teaspoon of the witch hazel to each tablespoonful of the infusion (average dose). Douching with an infusion of *lavender* flowers and leaves is also helpful. In severe cases the lavender infusion can also be given internally, at midday, in addition to the morning and evening dose of rose-hip infusion. The other part of the treatment is fasting and internal cleansing, making good use of the internal disinfecting, and mucus-expellent, powers of antiseptic herbs.

Mention should be made of the herbal cure of the Dandie Dinmont terrier, Ch. Peachems Wannie Blossom, owned by Mr. and Mrs. E. Stubbs, of Angmering, Sussex, the terrier being such a famous one. Three veterinary surgeons had seen this case and no hope of cure was given; a slight promise of recovery was given *only* if the bitch were operated on for the removal of the entire reproductive system. With herbs, and the bitch's own good health powers from her careful and natural rearing, she made a full recovery without operation.

MILK GLANDS TROUBLE. 'False' milk is often troublesome in bitches, also excess milk, following weaning. The former is generally met with in maiden bitches who produce milk at the times when, if mated, they would have been having a litter; however, brood bitches also can develop this 'false' milk when they have not

Ailments and Their Treatments

been mated. The treatment for this trouble is exactly the same as for metritis (which see), but with no external douching; and the treatment naturally being used in a much shorter form; for example, one day's fasting, followed by two or three days' milk-honey fluid diet. In this ailment it is more beneficial to use the milk in a sour state: in that way it becomes somewhat laxative; honey should still be given. The external treatment, in this trouble, is the bathing and massaging of the hot and inflamed milk glands with an infusion of *mint* leaves (common garden mint) or mint and *lettuce* leaves. An excellent alternative treatment is external bathing with *dock* and *elder* leaves. With this latter treatment I have had great success in curing mastitis in cows and goats. Internally, give twice daily in doses of two tablespoons a brew of *wood-sage*.

The same treatment should be followed for cases of excess milk in the dam following the removal of her weaned puppies. It is the over-early removal of a litter which is frequently the cause of the dam's excess milk: early sales often being the motive. The unnatural over-early weaning of puppies is one of the greatest causes of poor health among dogs; a well-bred brood bitch will be able to feed her litter until the puppies reach the age of seven to eight weeks, or longer; the puppy weaning not commencing before the fourth week, when fresh goat or cow milk can be given, soon followed by tree-barks flour, raw meat not being introduced into the diet until the fifth week.

MYXOMATOSIS. This terrible plague disease of rabbits so far has not harmed many dogs, even those which have eaten diseased rabbits. The best safeguard against all disease is healthful diet and internal disinfecting with garlic. If such disease should develop, treatment would be on hard-pad lines. (See Hard Pad.)

NERVOUSNESS. This is most frequently a hereditary or psychological ailment, best cured by careful breeding out through strong-nerved stock, and patient, intelligent handling of the nervous case. I, personally, have restored many a nervous animal to becoming a well-balanced, normal one—dog and horse.

Diet and herbs can, however, also play a helpful part.

Treatment. Short cleansing fasts. Use of leaf-plasma tablets (a great natural nerve tonic, very rich in iron and iodine); *seaweed*, *raisins*, egg yolks, molasses, *bran*, honey, *nettles* (used as a 'soup' for soaking of cereal biscuit meal), *wheat*-germ flakes or oil. In cases of true nerve sickness, *skullcap, rue, rosemary, vervain, peony*

145

Ailments and Their Treatments

root, *valerian, lime* blossom, *hops*, are all very helpful, given as a standard brew. Give seaweed.

OBESITY. This condition is generally more prevalent in bitches than in dogs, and is frequently of a glandular-sexual nature. Advanced obesity can be very serious, and is not only a certain cause of barrenness in bitches, but also a cause of premature death. An abnormal accumulation of fatty tissue is not merely a harbourer of toxic accumulations, but also puts great pressure on the blood system which has to pump its way through the semi-diseased (fatty) areas of the body. Great muscular development is very different from flabby fat, and when the condition of an animal is being judged in the show ring, due merit should be given to muscular development and there should be penalization of fatness. Most dogs are shown far too fat; a dog by nature and natural conformation being a lean creature, active and speedy of foot.

A corrective and very laxative diet is the main method for the internal breaking down of fatty tissue, the diet to be interspaced with short fasts of from two to three days on a diet of water only, with a daily *senna* laxative dose, of approximately two senna pods for an average-size dog. This will clear away fatty substances dissolved during treatment. External improvement must be largely regulated by abundant exercise, the exercise becoming increasingly strenuous as body improvement takes place. Encourage swimming in river or sea.

Castration of male and spaying of female animals, because they interfere with normal rhythm of the body and normal glandular health, create obesity and shorten life.

Treatment. A daily dose of an infusion of *rosemary* herb. The daily use of *parsley* and *dandelion* on the meat feed, together with daily dose of *seaweed* powder, because of its tonic effect on the glandular system. Starchy food should be greatly restricted, and to every half pound of whole-grain cereal used, one handful of raw bran should be added. Feed finely grated raw cabbage and onion mixed into the food and let raw and cooked carrots replace at least a quarter of the starchy cereal ration. Bitches and stud dogs should be allowed to lead normal sex lives, for lack of this is the commonest cause of the prevalent fatness seen among pet dogs and bitches.

PARALYSIS. This is not necessarily a distemper sequela, paralysis, especially of the hindquarters, often attacking young and aged

Ailments and Their Treatments

dogs. The trouble is caused by pressure on the roots of the nerves in a limb, or a group of muscles, or pressure on, or other interference with, the brain or the spinal cord itself; in the case of paralysis of the hindquarters, constipation may be the cause; a serious blow or fall can also bring on paralysis, as also can worm infestation. Paralysis of the hindquarters is a fairly common hereditary ailment of the dachshund and Pekinese breeds. But excellent results have been obtained with treatment. Indeed, hundreds of cases, many of them condemned as incurable, have been restored to full normal health.

Treatment. See Chorea. The *skullcap* infusion should be replaced by one of *sage* leaves. Give also *grape* juice. Externally, an infusion of *mustard* seed, one teaspoon of seed to one cup of boiling water, should be massaged twice daily into the paralysed areas. Mustard powder can be used in place of seed, same quantities; merely dissolve in boiling water and apply warm.

In my many years of veterinary work my most spectacular cure was with a case of paralysis—a pedigree Swaledale ewe with total paralysis of the hind legs of three months' duration. The ewe had become paralysed during the Great Snow of 1947; being especially valuable, she had been kept alive to await my expected visit to the farm—Kitley Farm, Arkengarthdale, Yorkshire. The limbs were cold and lifeless and covered with 'bed' sores. The exact canine paralysis treatment as given here was prescribed. In ten days of treatment the ewe was standing; in three weeks she was running so swiftly that she could no longer be caught for administering her medical treatment. The paralysis has never returned and the ewe has since given birth to one of the best lambs in the flock. In Arkengarthdale she is known as 'the miracle ewe'.

There comes to me from the same district, Swaledale, one of those 'dramatic' veterinary reports which make my herbal work seem worthwhile, and I am therefore persuaded to include the cure herewith in the text, as it is concerned with paralysis. From Mrs. Gladys Hutchinson, Helaugh, Richmond, North Yorkshire: 'I know you will be pleased to hear that a policeman all the way from Yarm brought a black Labrador bitch for me to treat by your method and thereby save, for the vets said that no more could be done for her. The police at Reeth told him to bring the bitch here, where your herbal methods are used. It had paralysis of the back legs. I did all that your treatment said, and in a

147

Ailments and Their Treatments

week had the Labrador walking and going out rabbiting with my husband, in fact I could not believe it myself. The policeman said he was going to take it straight to the vets to show them the dog that would have had a grave if it had not been for herbal treatment. He wishes to thank you.'

PIGMENTATION, FAULTY. Many dogs suffer from faulty pigmentation; this is especially true of specific breeds, and notably the imported ones.

The most unusual body parts for faulty pigmentation are nose, eye rims, toenails. Light noses, however, should not be penalized in the imported breeds during the winter months, for very often such is but the protective snow-blending colour of Nature, e.g. Samoyeds (Arctic); Afghans, light-coated (Afghanistan); Finnish spitz (Finland); Golden Retrievers and Borzois (Russia), may all quite correctly develop light noses during those months when their native countries would be experiencing snow.

Treatment. Where pigmentation is truly faulty, the quickest and well-proved remedy is *seaweed*, given in powder form, increasing by twice the normal daily tonic dose of seaweed. It is outstanding for the dark pigment that it produces. Also helpful are: finely chopped *watercress* and *mustard* and *cress*, *molasses*, *grape* juice, *raisins*.

PNEUMONIA, PLEURISY, BRONCHITIS. These lung ailments are often a complication of distemper. A typical pneumonia case will be seen breathing rapidly, with mouth kept closed.

These ailments properly treated can be cured as surely as canine distemper, and likewise usually run a course of three weeks.

Treatment. A first need is strict fasting in order to cleanse the body of toxins accumulated. It is the strenuous cleansing efforts of the body which are the main cause of the very high fever found in canine lung disorders and which are not an unfavourable condition. Second need is the use of antiseptic herbs, especially *garlic* and *eucalyptus*.

The action of garlic on the lungs is a remarkable one: it has been praised throughout the ages as a tuberculosis cure, and even in this modern time of artificial chemical medicine it is given credit as such. Recently the daily papers have published reports of work done by the Russian, Professor Thokin, of Toms University, in regard to tuberculosis, he having prepared a serum from onions and garlic which will kill tuberculosis bacilli after only five minutes' treatment. (At last the production of a harmless serum! And one not derived from the body fluids of artificially diseased and tortured animals.) Thirdly, there comes the strengthening and soothing of the body, especially the nerves, through the feeding of that miraculous product of Nature—*honey*—which substance, in pneumonia treatment, even at a time of high fever, can be made into honey balls and fed to the dog or pushed down the throat; the honey will give great relief to the inflamed throat. Three drops of oil of *eucalyptus* can be added twice daily to the honey balls. Finally, the provision of abundant fresh air, which is as essential to a pneumonia case as is water to a gastritis case, although orthodox medicine usually places more importance on much warmth than on fresh air. And the orthodox, in order to keep the sick dog 'warm and free from draughts'—being the way in which that common ruling is usually expressed—keep windows closed, and the dog is thereby ignorantly, and cruelly, deprived of the air which its panting lungs crave. The nasal passages can be kept open by the use of inhalants such as *eucalyptus*, *camphor*, *thyme*, in form of essential oils. All are rather strong for the dog, therefore use only one or two drops mixed well into lanoline and then pressed up the nostrils. These oils are very effective in cases of congested lungs. The throat and chest should then be frictioned with a lotion of one teaspoon eucalyptus to two tablespoons water. A few drops of eucalyptus can also be given twice daily on a small piece of cube sugar or on honey, pushed down the throat.

Having given an outline of things to do in pneumonia treatment, it is also necessary for me to mention a few of the things *not* to do. Firstly, the rigid avoidance of all chemical drugs, especially those of the sulphonamide group. The rapid 'cure' that such drugs often produce is no real cure, it is merely suppression of the symptoms of pneumonia through violent interference of the drug in the body's cleansing efforts; such false healing provides ideal soil for the breeding, later, of tubercular bacteria. (Note present-day tuberculosis increase.) Secondly, the refraining from the giving of all the usual stimulants so commonly prescribed in the treatment of pneumonia.

An excellent medicine is made from the skins of washed *lemons*, three lemons to one and one-half pints cold water. Bring to boil for three minutes. When cooled to tepid, restore the juice of the lemons. Sweeten with one tablespoon honey. Add two inches solid

Ailments and Their Treatments

stick *Spanish liquorice*; dissolve well. The liquorice dissolved in this brew will then have its medicinal properties further enhanced. Also thick, pure honey rolled into balls and placed in the mouth or pressed down the throat gives nourishment, removes throat soreness and, like the liquorice, produces expectoration.

In the treatment kennel the air can be kept sweet and moist by using a steam kettle, a few drops of such a substance as eucalyptus oil or Vapex being added to each pint of water poured into the kettle. The freshening effect this has on the atmosphere is remarkable, and is highly appreciated by the dog. Elecampane herb and pine needles can also be used for inhalation by steam vapour.

The mouth and throat should be cleansed three times daily with lemon water, also the nose thoroughly washed or syringed out with the lemon water, while the body must be internally disinfected with *garlic*, which exerts a remarkable healing effect on the mucous membranes.

If this treatment is carried out faithfully, the dog will remain strong and will be found to be easily cured of this complication. But if the treatment is not fully and sufficiently followed, then there is a danger of the dread oedema of the lungs, brought about by the weakening of the heart on its left side and its subsequent failure to drive the venous blood through the lungs. Blood-filled fluid begins to pass through the nostrils, 'squelching' sounds can be heard in the lungs, and death takes place, the blood then flowing out through the mouth.

Let me repeat, such a happening is unusual, and is very rare if the case has been correctly treated.

Note. A dog with complications of the lungs *craves* fresh air. Fresh air at such a time is of far greater importance than food.

POISONING. The commonest poisons with which a dog is likely to come into contact are as follows (their neutralizing agents—antidotes—are bracketed with them): Strychnine—in vermin exterminators—(permanganate of potash in solution, about a saltspoonful to half a pint of tepid water). Phosphorus—in rat poison, matchheads—(soda water and milk of magnesia). Crude stove paraffin (stiff dose of salad oil to mix with the paraffin and cause its removal through the bowels). White lead—from paint, etc.—(Epsom salts in solution: about one teaspoon to one cupful tepid water).

Treatment. The general treatment is the same for all poisons,

150

Ailments and Their Treatments

only differing in the antidotes to be used. First there must be rapid removal of all possible poison by the aid of an emetic, the best of which is a piece of washing-soda, the size of a quarter-piece for an average-size dog, pushed well down the throat; this will induce almost immediate vomiting. Failing soda, common salt should be used: a stiff dose of two teaspoons in a small cupful of tepid water being the general dose. After the emetic has been given, the next principle is laxative treatment to clear the bowels of the poison. The best treatment is drenching with one of the natural aperient waters; failing this, then *senna* must be made quickly by scalding about seven pods with boiling water, allowing to stand for a few minutes, then crushing the pods to extract all moisture and reducing to blood heat by the addition of a little cold water. The dog must then be fasted for at least two to three days to allow the body, freed from the task of food digestion, to exert all of its energies on the removal of the irritant poisons, and also in the mere maintenance of life. Laxatives should be given night and morning, and the antidotes should be discontinued after the first day. The fast should be one of water only. If the dog has retained life up to the third day, then healing treatment can be commenced. Whether a dog is to live or to die, following intake of poison, largely depends on the dog's previous health record. A well-reared healthy animal will have great natural reserves of body energy with which to expel the poison from the body; and also there will be no danger of heart failure, which is the commonest cause of death in poisoning cases. Honey should be given from the very first hour of poisoning: for its heart and nerve restorative properties, also laxative and alkaline properties, internal healing powers, are all of the greatest value. Lumps of thick honey, about the size of a 5p piece—average dose—should be pushed down the throat four or five times per day during the first stages of the treatment. Following the fast, a recuperative diet should consist of three meals per day of one cupful of *slippery-elm* food (tree-barks blend) mixed with honey and milk. More can be given if the dog appears hungry: three to four cupfuls of the mixture for a large-sized dog, as required. The slippery elm acts as an internal poultice, soothing and healing the inflamed lining of stomach and intestines. After an average of three days on such fluid diet, the fluid can be thickened with flaked barley for the midday and evening meals, but no other food should be given for at least seven days, as the body will be in no fit state to deal with other foods. I should mention the use, also, of my own formula medicine, the leaf-plasma tablets, which are highly alkaline in their action, and are so wonderfully nerve restorative.

There is one thing of special importance in phosphorus poisoning (which poisoning may well be caused through the eating of matchheads—a common habit in young puppies—or from rat and mice exterminators): all fats must be withheld during treatment, in order to keep extra work from the liver which is the organ most usually affected in this type of poisoning, and also fats are an extra-harmful mixture with phosphorus. All milk given must be skimmed. In phosphorus poisoning the dog develops an ungovernable thirst, the intake of water each time being followed by severe vomiting which is very exhausting. However, I am of the opinion that it is wrong to withhold water, and at the usual meal hours, three times daily, the dog should be allowed to drink its fill of water. *Rue* is an ancient and famed poison antidote. The plant is crushed and rolled into pills.

An infusion of *hyssop* plant given morning and evening is highly effective as a remedial agent in all forms of poisoning. Foxes are said to seek out this plant when poisoned. Neat *witch hazel*, a tablespoon three times daily, given with the hyssop, and given alone at midday, is invaluable on account of its healing powers.

I have had two personal experiences of poisoning among my own Afghan hounds; in both cases very large amounts of poison were taken. The first case was an Afghan bitch, given a half-pint drench of stove paraffin in error, from a bottle which should by rights have held aperient water. Treated as instructed above, she fully recovered in ten days and has had perfect health ever since (this was the Best-in-Show winning bitch, Turkuman Wild Kashmiri Iris). The second case was of phosphorus rat-poisoning in an Afghan dog. Many pieces of bread spread thickly with rat poison had been eaten. The dog was the equally well-known Turkuman Mogul Rose-tree; no one thought he could recover.

I feel strongly that the making of phosphorus vermin poisons should be prohibited, that terrible internal burning is too cruel even for the vermin for which they are intended. Vermin-poisons manufacturers should be made to witness animals in the terrible death throes from their products.

RHEUMATISM. In damp climates rheumatism is a quite frequent

Ailments and Their Treatments

ailment of dogs, especially aged ones. Only the dampness is not wholly responsible: the body first has to be in an unhealthy condition to produce this condition of rheumatism or arthritis. A tendency to joint ailments also can be inherited; but as with most hereditary ailments, can be bred out by Natural Rearing. Canine rheumatism is found most frequently in shoulders and chest, or back and loins—where it is called lumbago. The feet are sometimes affected. In the limbs lameness often develops. The only certain preventative of rheumatism is: correct rearing on a raw-foods diet, with provision of good, dry housing, and especially the avoidance of sour, urine-saturated kennel runs; and also providing all the sunlight that the dogs themselves desire.

Internal Treatment. Internal cleansing with antiseptic herbs, especially *garlic*; honey is also an important remedy, its alkaline properties reducing the acid deposits of rheumatism. An infusion of *parsley* leaves, or fed raw, finely minced, is excellent, especially when the ailment is chronic. Parsley alone has cured even severe cases of rheumatism and arthritis. Also give as much *nettle* as possible, for above all other plants it has the power to dissolve uric acid crystals and therefore gives much relief in rheumatic ailments. Nettles should be gathered with scissors, as the leafage stings the hands, then plunged into boiling water for a few minutes, using very little water; they are then ready for use, mixed into the cereal feed. I have prepared tablets of nettle with seaweed and *comfrey*. Comfrey is a proved remedy for rheumatism and arthritis.

External Treatment. Massage with lotion made from an infusion of *seaweed* and *thyme*, equal parts, standard infusion. Apply warm. Give also, on the meat, finely chopped green leaves of *celery*, also a dessertspoon of celery seed. Miss D. Mills, The Kennels, Dawlish, Devon, reported: 'I have cured an Irish Setter—after only three weeks' treatment—of prolonged and acute rheumatism, by your herbal treatment. The dog was so ill he could not stand and the orthodox treatment could do nothing more for him.'

RINGWORM. This fungus disease is distinguished by circular patches on any part of the body, often on the face. The hair falls. Treat as for Mange.

RUBARTH DISEASE. (This is contagious hepatitis; see Hepatitis.)

SCALDS. Many small dogs, especially toys and terrier breeds,

Ailments and Their Treatments

get under the feet of their owners when they are carrying boiling water, and get badly scalded. I learned a burns-scald treatment from peasants of the Sierra Nevada mountains, Spain, which gives remarkable results. Bathe the injured area first with pure vinegar, then spread honey thickly over the area, ten minutes later. Keep applying dressings of honey until all burning pain ceases, then bandage lightly with cotton cloths over a dressing of honey to exclude air. Long-haired dogs must be clipped before applying the honey: they would lose their burnt or scalded hair anyway. If the dog tries to tear off the bandaging, he must wear a broad collar of cardboard to restrict movement of his head. Another excellent and proved burns-scalds remedy is raw *potato*. Pulp up raw potato and apply the juicy pulp to the area, or the potato can be finely grated and the juice expressed by pressing through cheesecloth. Then if none of these remedies are available, there is a cure learned from the natives of Hawaii. Place the injured area under tepid water, and keep under water, excluding all air, for at least one hour, until the burning pain ceases. Application of egg whites is curative.

SCURF. Presence of much scurf indicates excess mucus in the system. Also lack of exercise in fresh air will create greasy skin and thus scurf.

Treatment. This is both internal and external. Internal is dependent upon diet. Cut down on milk and starches. Feed, instead, cooked, minced *carrot*. Feed minced *watercress*. Externally friction with a brew of *meadowsweet*. Also the hair treatment for Baldness (see this chapter) can be used with advantage.

SEASON, DELAYED OR FAULTY. (See Streptococcal Infection.) The simple cleansing treatment for 'strep' will restore normality to the reproductive organs. But it is necessary to advise that bitches of some breeds, especially the Oriental ones such as Afghans, Salukis, and Chows, are often only once yearly in season when in normal health. Give *raspberry* leaves, raw and minced, mixed with food, or as an infusion.

SENILITY. Senility in the dog and cat (also in humans) is caused largely by the daily feeding of cooked foods in place of the natural raw, and by lack of sufficient running exercise, causing the blood to lack oxygen and also the lungs and heart to degenerate. Today many dogs are declining in health from the age of seven years, and most of them have disordered kidneys from that age onwards. In the old days when dog rearing was more natural, dogs remained

Ailments and Their Treatments

in good health up to twenty years of age. I have met a number of dogs of such age owned by desert-roaming Bedouin Arabs and by Spanish peasants. In Granada, Spain, a market stall-holder had a spaniel aged twenty-four years, and Sunny Shay, Grandeur Afghans, New York, kept her Afghan, Champion Taj Akbaruu of Grandeur, to the age of twenty-two.

After fifteen years of N.R. in Switzerland, Miss Marjorie Pickance, La Tour de Peilz, Ct. Vaud, owner of the Kentony Pekinese, known throughout Switzerland for their great health (now retired from showing and breeding), writes to me: 'I have two stud dogs who are thirteen and look and behave as if they were about six, and a bitch of nearly fifteen. All are a tremendous credit to N.R. Most of the others are over ten. All these dogs are in wonderful condition and coat and seem to enjoy every minute of the day and every meal. No need to coax any of them to eat, we have always kept strictly to N.R. diet.'

Also in this book among the veterans (last photos) will be seen dogs from famous N.R. kennels in England. Saluki champion Knightellington Vandal is photographed after winning Best-in-Show at the Saluki Club Show of England, when aged nearly ten years. Saved by herbal medicine when his life was despaired of, he is reared and owned by the Misses Kean and Mackenzie, at their Ajman Kennels, Oxford. Country dogs, living free, unchained, hunting around, are notable for long life, as likewise are the dogs of gypsies and wandering Bedouins of the Arab lands. Such people commonly own dogs who live into their twentieth year and over, horses (and camels) of these natural people likewise are exceptionally long-lived. The United States Ch. Turkuman Nissim's Laurel, exported from my Turkuman Afghan kennel to Sol. M. Malkin and Sunny Shay, Grandeur Afghans, lived to the age of sixteen years, siring champions when aged fourteen, and winning Hound Groups when turned twelve years.

For longevity for *all* dogs, feed a *raw*-foods diet, as Nature intended for the dog, fox, wolf, etc. (Some wolves in the wild, recognizable by their battle scars by those who have seen them on the Turkish hills, attain thirty years of age.) Provide also sunlight and free-running exercise; and long life will be your dog's heritage.

SHOCK. When a dog or cat is suffering from shock, resulting from severe wounds in a fight or from car or other accidents, do not give solid food for twenty-four hours; give instead a teaspoon

Ailments and Their Treatments

of pure honey, liquefied by stirring in one-half teaspoon of brandy or wine. Then restore to normal food, beginning with one day on fluid milk-honey only.

SICKNESS, AND PROLONGED VOMITING. As with diarrhoea, sickness in the dog is usually either a rapid, natural cleansing of the body or a mere symptom of some other ailment: distemper, leptospirosis, hepatitis (see treatments, this chapter). Deliberate sickness is produced in the dog by eating of couch grass, which acts as an internal rake, scraping out mucus-embedded impurities. Prolonged frothy, yellow sickness needs treatment to sweeten the digestive system, and vomiting of food needs immediate fasting.

Treatment. Herbs to sweeten a sour digestive tract, cause of prolonged sickness, are, *peppermint*, *rosemary*, *thyme*, and tablets of vegetable charcoal. Make infusion of one or another of these herbs, and give to the fasting dog—dose, two tablespoons three times daily. In the dangerous vomiting of Stuttgart disease and some other ailments, grate raw *gentian* root preferably, or buy the powdered root. Roll the grated gentian into pills the size of a garden pea, using a mass of thick honey and flour to bind it. An average dog would require approximately twelve pills for a day's treatment. Fast the dog on lemon-water only during the gentian treatment.

Bitches in sound health often suffer from a slight nervous sickness during the first few weeks of the in-whelp period. This does not indicate ill health; merely give infusion of *raspberry* leaves and two or three charcoal tablets morning and night.

There is also sickness caused by nervous excitability, travel by car, ship, or plane. The greyhound breeds seem to be the most frequent sufferers from travel sickness. Animals prone to such sickness should be fasted for at least twelve hours before long journeys. At the time of travel they should be given balls of thick honey pressed down their throats; honey will settle the stomach nerves; or yet a better remedy is to mix tree-barks flour into the honey, one small teaspoon of flour to one heaped tablespoon thick honey. Dogs travel best on car floors rather than seats if they are bad travellers; however, car floors cannot be used during hot weather as they heat up and are harmful then to health.

SORE PADS, SPLIT PADS, ETC. Concrete roads, gravel paths, and flinty hillsides often injure the foot pads of dogs when they take much exercise over such surfaces. The normal surface for the dog is earth—grassland, sands, or rocks. The dogs of heavy build, such as Great Danes, Irish wolfhounds, Newfoundlands, etc., are the most prone to this trouble. Generally bad feet are also a sign of health decline; and attention, therefore, should be given to the diet, especially if the dog is overweight.

Treatment. Rest the dog from all exercise or work for several days, at least until the splits in the pads close up. Bathe the pads three times daily with a lotion made from boiled *potato* peelings, one large handful of peelings to one quart cold water, brought to a boil and simmered for ten minutes. Do not strain. Deep fissures should be treated with swabs of cotton soaked in a lotion made from *ivy* leaves. To every cupful of the ivy, add one dessertspoon of *witch hazel*. A dusting with fine oatmeal completes the treatment. At night soak the feet in *castor* oil and tie on cloths.

SPRAINS. These are usually caused by running over hard land, especially land rutted by ploughing, or landing badly from a high jump. With a sprain the dog limps badly and swelling often occurs.

Treatment. Resting and application of cold-water cloths packed around the limb. An old and effective horse remedy is to apply a paste made from whitening (whitewash) and cow dung. Spread thickly around the affected area and bandage lightly. The herbal remedies are *comfrey* or *mallow*. Make a standard infusion of either herb and bathe the injured area before applying bandages. Dog owners who live by the sea can stand the injured dog in the sea, or put the limb standing in a bucket of sea water for ten minutes or so. This is a very simple and effective cure, much used for valuable race-horses.

STERILITY. Animals which are habitually sterile may well be carriers of streptococcal bacteria or of leptospirosis or hepatitis. But mention should be made of the effect of diet on fertility. Modern diet greatly lacks the fertility vitamins, which are removed in modern milling, especially vitamins B and E. Sterility may also be caused by obesity (see Obesity).

Treatment. Place all sterile animals on a natural raw-foods diet (see N.R. diet chart, Chapter 1). Give leaf-extract tablets containing seaweed, nettle, etc., also give wheat-germ flakes and raw eggs. Natural, herbal aphrodisiacs are *balm*, mint (especially *wild water mint*), and the aromatics, *thyme, marjoram, sage*, and *fennel*. All should be given very finely chopped on the raw meat. Honey also aids fertility, and young *maize* (corn) cobs, given grated on a

Ailments and Their Treatments

vegetable grater. Grated raw *almonds* are a splendid fertility aid, especially for male animals; mix the almonds with the cereal. Feed, also, raw eggs. Feed liquorice to females. (See photo and caption of the Bullmastiff bitch, Wyaston Elizabeth Tudor, this book.)

STREPTOCOCCAL INFECTION. The one and only cause of streptococcal infections and losses, as with distemper, is faulty rearing and over-commercialism. I have often given the opinion that a large percentage of present-day dog breeders would happily feed their dogs on a diet of sawdust if they could get away with it!

The wish for cheap, quickly prepared foods and medicines, and utter neglect of kennel hygiene, with horrible overcrowding, sour earth and urine-soaked wooden buildings typify dog rearing today in most countries, and dogs will continue to suffer from 'plague' diseases until the simple laws of natural, clean, and kindly dog rearing become common to the majority of kennels. Nature Rearing has already been put into world-wide practice, and in kennels, where once not a single litter had been reared in years, now litters are being reared easily, the stock showing a high standard of health. I have also met with many half-hearted kennelmen who allege that they are rearing on natural, healthful lines, but who are continuing to keep their stock overcrowded and under-exercised: not all the medicines—herbal or otherwise—nor the most perfect of diets will be able to maintain normal health in such cases. I am not at all impressed with kennels keeping anything over twenty dogs. I cannot understand the mentality of such kennel owners. Is it that they think that in having large numbers the law of averages makes the breeding of a champion the more certain? But how different are the true facts as to the breeding of champions: again and again it will be found that it is the 'little' kennel owner who breeds the champions, and the other 'big' kennels which buy up their winning stock—and often lose through disease, latent in their kennels, the new-purchased stock.

It will be appropriate here to quote from a remarkable agricultural booklet, sent to me by one of my veterinary clients, Miss C. D. Wilson, of Ludlow, and which upholds in every instance all that I have been stating and writing for so many years on the subject of canine rearing and medicine. It is *Re-Fertilization of a Large Wiltshire Farm by Compost*, by F. Sykes;[1] its writer stresses

[1] Friend Sykes, author of *Modern Humus Farming* and *Food, Farming and the Future* (Faber and Faber).

that healthy soil is the root of all health and of disease prevention and cure, that all chemicals both in soil treatment and food materials should be strictly avoided, and likewise use of all vaccine and similar remedies. A case is quoted of a thoroughbred mare which developed contagious abortion, and whose destruction was advised by an 'eminent veterinarian'; the mare was subjected to natural medicine methods and made a perfect recovery (typical of numerous cases of streptococcal infection in bitches, which cases, removed to clean kennel runs [grass-sown], correctly dieted, sufficiently exercised, have made perfect recoveries and have whelped and nursed perfectly normal litters, the puppies of which have grown up into disease-free adults—this, from bitches tested for presence of b.h.s., and found to be 'infected').

To quote Mr. Sykes: '. . . our most valuable thoroughbred mare contracted the dangerous disease—contagious abortion. An eminent veterinarian advised her destruction. I declined the advice and determined a treatment of my own, which was to turn the mare out into a large paddock where no horse stock had been grazed, where artificial manures had never been used, and where she was condemned to live for two years eating practically nothing but grass. At the end of this period she was examined by a competent vet and declared clean. She was mated and artificially inseminated; she later proved in foal, and subsequently bred over the next seven years four valuable foals, she herself living to the ripe age of 21 years. Here was my first attempt to cure an allegedly incurable disease by giving the creature nothing but grass-grown land where artificial manures had never been applied, in other words Nature's food from humus-filled land.'

The writer then goes on to describe how large-scale disease came to the farm (through the usual causes which are the same source of disease in dog kennels). Again I quote from this booklet: 'We bought valuable cattle and put them on land which was couch-ridden and very infertile, and the ability of which to sustain life was so low that food of every kind had to be brought from elsewhere to augment the supply of the poor herbage. The heavy stocking and treading began to develop other troubles and, as always on dirty, foul, neglected land, disease of every kind began to show itself in the cattle to the pre-war value of over £2,000. The veterinary service could help us but little. As is usual, the course followed had to be devised by the farmer. We decided to plough up the whole

Ailments and Their Treatments

750 acres. We determined to try now home-grown food, especially avoiding all factory compound foods and concentrates. Above all to apply artificials nowhere. And after seven years of heart-breaking toil, with the added difficulties of war-time (1) completely rid the farm of disease; (2) built up a large herd of home-bred, attested dairy cattle, tubercle-free for over three years now, and of a soundness of constitution to all critical appearances such that no expert would believe that any scourge had ever visited the farm, and (3) as each succeeding generation of young stock is born we have unmistakable evidence of still greater stamina and endurance.'

The (3) result is of special importance to dog breeders, for likewise in dog breeding, with each generation of natural-reared stock improved health is a natural and positive result—greater size, bone, hair growth, and general disease resistance.

Concerning all this, Mrs. Doxford, the cocker spaniel judge and breeder, Broomleaf Cockers, Ewshot, Surrey, has reported: 'I am rearing my fifth generation of N.R.—natural reared—stock now; and their disease resistance is amazing, as is their growth and condition. What I think is even more satisfactory (to both you and me) is that young stock sold from these kennels have come through epidemics in their new owners' kennels, *unscathed*; whereas the other stock has succumbed; the other stock of course not having been reared by natural methods.'

In the latter end of his leaflet, in his summing-up, Mr. Sykes, concerning disease prevention and the appalling record of disease rife in the world today, writes as follows: 'Then is there no hope for mankind? Yes, there is one hope—disease. It may teach us the mistakes we should avoid. The continued use of artificials is the first mistake, for it produces food of diminishingly efficient feeding value for both man and beast, and is reducing vitality so low that resistance to the malign bacteria of disease is becoming less. Notwithstanding, the Ministry of Health can be liquidated in a very short time. The second mistake is the feeding of concentrated cakes and meals, the by-products of the soap and oil industries—yet more of the powerful vested interests. They are unnatural foods and are fed to cattle and poultry to stimulate the production of unnatural quantities of meat, milk, eggs, and poultry meat. I have cured disease in animals by cutting-out the feeding of factory-made concentrates and substituting such foods as oats, peas, beans, and grass, grown on the farm on humus-sufficient fertile

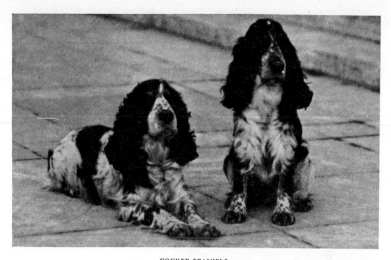

COCKER SPANIELS

Cocker Spaniels. French field and bench champions. Betty Butterworth (Coigny), 306, W. 18th St., N.Y.C., New York, a friend of the author, has raised some of France's most outstanding spaniels and has followed N.R. for years.

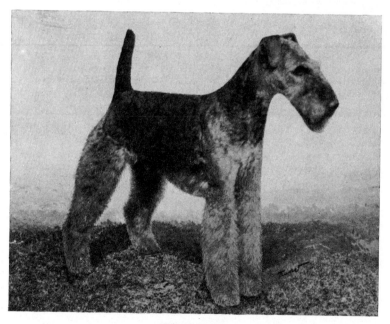

AIREDALE TERRIER

Mrs. M. Harmsworth, Bath, Somerset. Bred by Mrs. Harmsworth, Bengal Airedales, exported to H. Florsheim, Chicago. Acclaimed by experts as a model of his breed, this terrier was Best Airedale two years in succession at the Airedale Club Show, U.S.A. (*Photo: Thurse*)

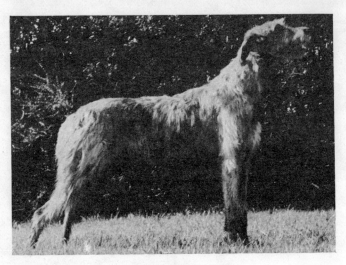

CHAMPION BRANWEN LUATH

(American, French, Spanish and Italian Champion) Irish Wolfhound. Mrs. Cynthia Madigan,
Branwen Kennels, Villa Levona, San Sebastian, Spain. Luath won Best in Show, Madrid, 1965.
Mrs. Madigan has made breed history in many breeds, including Salukis and Afghans. The Princess
of Afghanistan bought a Branwen Afghan. A long-time friend of the author, Mrs. Madigan,
like the author, insists on whole foods and remedies for her children as well as her dogs.

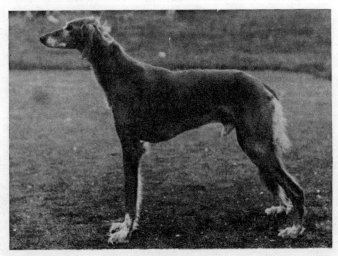

CHAMPION KNIGHTELLINGTON VANDAL

Saluki. Misses P. Kean and E. Mackenzie, Ajman Salukis and Afghans, Hornsway House, Oxford.
Vandal in veteran class won Best in Show, English Saluki Club Championship Show, when nearly
ten years old. 'Our feeding and management is still 100 per cent N.R.' (*Photo: C. M. Cooke*)

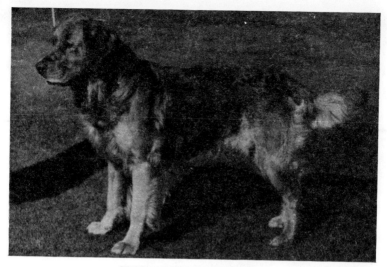

CHAMPION ULWIN VINTAGE OF YELME

Golden Retriever. Mrs. M. K. Wentworth-Smith, Yelme Kennels, Northwold, Norfolk. Mrs. Wentworth-Smith is one of England's greatest judges of gundogs, and with the help of the skilled kennel management of Miss Eva Todd, the Yelmes represent the best in Natural Rearing. Vintage is a son of the great Ch. Dernar of Yelme. Vintage has won Best in Show at G.R. Breed Championship Shows, 1959, 1963 (Jubilee), 1968 and Best Dog, 1969. Also Best of Breed, Crufts, 1962. A truly remarkable record for a dog also famed as a field worker. He descends straight from the first known Golden Retrievers, when known as 'Russian Retrievers". (*Photo: C. M. Cooke*)

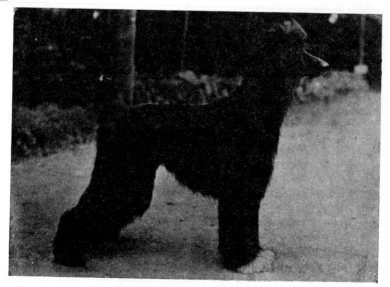

CHAMPION TURKUMAN NISSIM'S LAUREL

Afghan Hound, Sol. M. Malkin and Sunny Shay, Grandeur Kennels, Long Island, N.Y. The author took over the hound's care when he was condemned by veterinary surgeons as a case of incurable rickets. Herbal medicine and N.R. restored him to such health that he was Best of Breed at the American Afghan Show, Best of Breed and of Hound Group, Westminster 1950 (*Photo: Tauskey*)

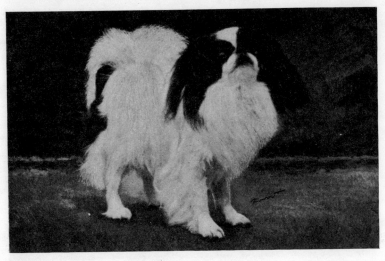

CHAMPION CAROLINE OF RIU GU

Japanese Spaniel. Mrs. Eileen A. Crauford, Glebe House, Wormington, Broadway, Worcs., has reared generations of healthy Riu Gus on N.R.; many have become champions. (*Photo: B. Thuse*)

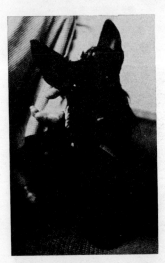

BIMBO

Scottish terrier. Pet of the Gerhard Gunther family, Loerrach, Switzerland. Read in Chapter 6, under 'Mange', how Mrs. Helen Balk-Roesch, also of Loerrach, saved Bimbo from destruction, using herbal treatment.

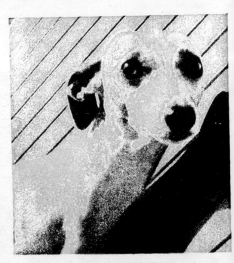

LAGUNA LADY LIGHTFOOT

Whippet. Mrs. L. Gut, In der Ey 27, Wangen bei Olten, Switzerland. This beautiful whippet is another triumph for herbs. In March 1961, after failure of orthodox treatments for Follicular Mange, and College examination, and diagnosis (England)—'hereditary F. Mange, and at least one year of arsenic treatment required,' herbal treatment from this book was tried. By July 1961 the whippet was *cured*; Bill Siggers, the judge, found her in 'excellent condition'. The cure was complete and the whippet has won C.C.s in Italy and has bred many champions.

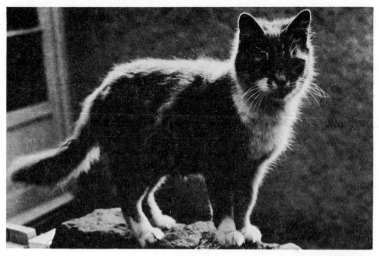

KIT-KAT GROWN

At time of previous edition she was a kitten. Owned and photographed by well-known photographer Powell Jones, Gendros, Swansea, S. Wales, she is a good example of N.R. and finds her own herbs in the garden. Powell Jones has used and recommended N.R. for years. He previously lost three Alsatians from Hard-pad on orthodox rearing and treatment, then saved his white Alsatian Zante by herbal methods when Hard-pad again developed. (*Photo: Powell Jones*)

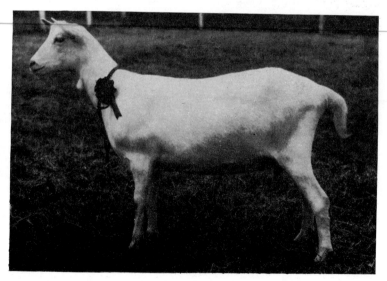

CHAMPION FOXLEY LUATH

British Saanen Goat. Mrs. Leslie Harrison, Grove House, Tarporley, Cheshire. Winner of Holmes Peglar Trophy 1961, Royal Dairy Show (a supreme honour of the British Goat World), 11 Breed Challenge Certificates, 5 milking awards. Here photographed as a goatling. Francia is a second generation of N.R. Mrs. Harrison was so impressed with N.R. for her dogs that she applied the method to her goats. When many were poisoned from nearby weed-spraying with dangerous chemicals, herbal treatment saved them. Princess was left out in the snow by mistake after kidding, she got mastitis, and was completely cured by herbal treatment, and her udder is perfect. (*Photo: J. E. L. Mayes*)

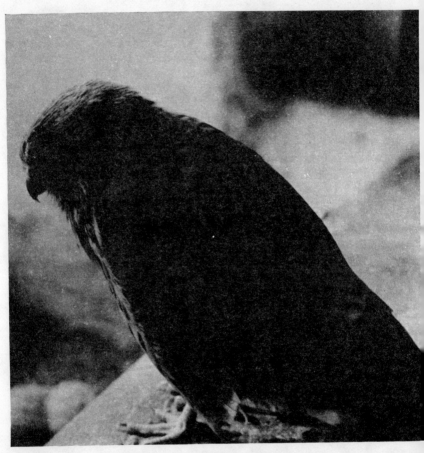

TURKUMAN GLOBE-THISTLE 'ARTEMISIA'

A young hen hawk, from a pair raised almost from hatching, by the author. Nature-reared, able to live wild
and trained to return home. Their story, with many photos, will be told in a short book by Juliette de Baïracli
Levy, *Hawks in a Carob Tree*. When very young the hawks had dangerous dysentery; their food was always
natural raw, but it was difficult to find their true insect and rodent diet. Cured by a diet of Tree-barks food
(as described in this book for weaning and treatment of dysentery). (*Photo: Rafik Bairacli*)

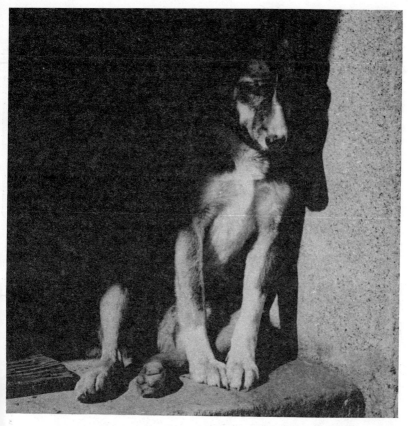

TAKE PROPER CARE OF YOUR WATCHDOG!

Every animal owner knows that proper housing and care is well worth while, not only for the animals themselves but also in his own financial interests. However, there is one domestic animal for which there is usually no care or even pity: the watchdog. Day and night the poor creature is the prisoner of a chain which is usually too short. In summer, when the sun beats down on his kennel, he desperately tries to find some shade. Droppings accumulate around his kennel since they are not removed and the dog cannot go anywhere else because of the chain. There is nobody to deliver him from vermin which is often a plague. Even if this is done occasionally—it is so easy nowadays—nobody thinks of the vermin-infested kennel which should also be cleaned out and disinfected with boiling water. The watchdog is often given stale food in a dish that is rarely cleaned. It is often forgotten that his drinking water needs changing: 'He hasn't emptied his bowl yet.' The worst time, however, for the watchdog is winter. Damp and cold penetrate through cracks in the walls of his kennel. Only too often there is no proper dry straw bedding and even more often no sacking at the entrance of the kennel to keep out draughts. Sometimes the unfortunate animal pleads for a few hours' freedom from the chain, but all in vain. (*Copyright: The World Federation for the Protection of Animals, P.O.B. 5061, 8022, Zurich, Switzerland*)

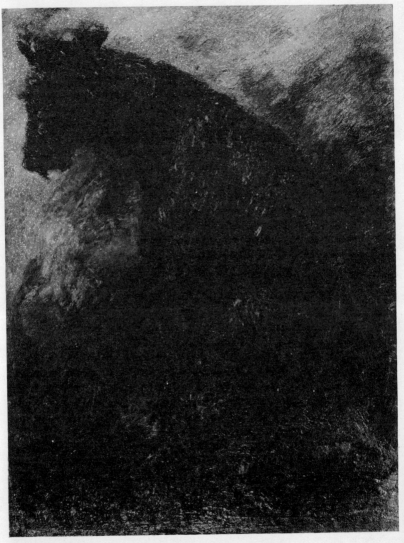

'LE CHIEN' BY GEORGES BRUNON

This painting is reproduced here because it is the *true* dog, savage, proud, ever watchful, and above all strong and healthy. This boarhound of the French forests is typical of the work of Brunon, whose nature paintings, especially of beasts and birds, are famed far beyond his native France. Brunon is a long-time friend of the the author and gave her this reproduction of his painting for use in her book, because he himself believes in herbs and nature diet.

Ailments and Their Treatments

land.' (Here should be mentioned that the by-products of soap and other industries are in use also in the canine world. The dried meat in use in popular dog foods is often the residue from soap factories, animal material from which all fat has been extracted by means of caustics, in soap manufacture—the harmfulness of such 'food' to the canine stomach and intestines can well be imagined.)

To continue from the agricultural treatise: 'Two difficulties presented themselves. (1) Farmers will not cease to use artificial fertilizers for their land, because they have been taught by clever propaganda over a long period of time, that it is more profitable to use them for crop production than keeping and relying upon livestock. . . . (2) Farmers will continue the use of factory concentrates for their cattle feeding, because again skilled propaganda has driven into their heads that they can produce neither milk nor meat without them. It does not begin to occur to one farmer in a thousand that the prevalence of contagious abortion, tubercular and other ills of their livestock may be brought about by the use of artificials on the land, or the use of the concentrated cakes fed to cows. . . . And so disease will come. Come? It is already here, everywhere in abundance. There are few disease-free herds in this country. Foot-and-mouth is periodically rampant; tuberculosis is as common as the dawn of day; Johne's disease and barrenness are rife everywhere. It is estimated on reliable data that eighty per cent of dairy cattle passing through the market are diseased in one way or another. The milking life of the average cow is now reduced to two and a half years. Is the Ministry of Agriculture worried? Yes, indeed they are. Remedies? Oh, yes, vaccines and veterinary panels. But why not start at the bottom, in the soil itself? Hush! No one has ever thought of that. *In officialdom you must never go to the root cause of disease. That is a most unprofessional approach*' (the italics are my stressing—J. de B.-L.).

As in agriculture, the canine world is faced with misleading propaganda largely sponsored by vaccine and chemical manufacturers, and the equally mischievous advertising of the Ministry of Health, with its stress on the importance of diphtheria inoculation and the 'fine' results obtained (such propaganda is becoming increasingly necessary because members of the armed forces in World War II, having witnessed the deleterious effect of army vaccinations on their own health, are insisting that their children be kept free of such unhygienic and unnatural practices).

Ailments and Their Treatments

Then, as with the farmers, there is the laziness of dog breeders. Correct rearing takes much time. In natural diet alone it requires far more care and thought than the general orthodox-feeding method—a method which is fit only for the raising of those fat semi-diseased beasts, swine—of over-boiling supplies of meat, pouring the resultant liquid over white hound meal with its percentage of soap-factory by-product meat fibre, and feeding both meat and greasy white-cereal biscuit together at one meal, and expecting good health to result! (Little wonder that tapeworm remedies are in great demand, and eczema and hysteria cures!) Proper feeding takes much care and time and planning; the preparation of the daily ration for each dog, of raw finely chopped green food—a health essential—takes time, the herbs have to be gathered, let alone prepared for use. Raw meat takes longer to cut up than cooked—for the latter is partly disintegrated flesh; the whole-grain cereal dishes need careful preparation; and ample supply of fresh unpasteurized milk is required—for dried milk is one of the most deadly and mischievous foods offered to dogs, and especially to young puppies, etc. That is why I state very emphatically that it is not possible for good health to be maintained in any kennel where the number of inmates is overlarge. Cattle can be kept in herds of fair size: they get most of their own foods through grazing—it is merely necessary to ensure that their pasture is healthy; but dogs must have all of their food fed to them by man—except for occasional rabbits which they may take themselves; and, furthermore, dogs quickly foul and sour the premises where they are kept and the ground on which they take exercise—cattle are mainly beneficial to the land. *Overcrowding, wrong feeding, neglectful rearing—especially where sufficient exercise is concerned—use of chemicals and vaccines in canine medicine with the subsequent health degeneration are the root causes of present-day prevalence of canine b.h.s. disease.* The remedy for its prevention and cure lies in the hands of the breeders.

And now to go on to streptococcal disease itself. It is absurd to take the mere presence of streptococcal bacteria as being proof of the presence of the disease, especially when it should be remembered that streptococcal bacteria are among the most widely distributed and the most common of all bacteria of the body, and are to be found wherever pus is present—in surface wounds, eczema sores, for instance. The veterinary profession have themselves rightly

162

Ailments and Their Treatments

pointed out that beta haemolytic streptococcus bacteria are themselves incapable of producing an acute condition in the body without the interference of other more toxic bacteria; therefore, as yet, we have no evidence to prove that the b.h.s. bacteria solely are responsible for sterility, abortion, fading of new-born puppies, death of weaned puppies, skin ailments, all of which are attributed to b.h.s. merely on the unsubstantial evidence that these bacteria have been taken in swabs from all such infected organs, bodies, or areas. The majority of the above symptoms can more generally be attributed to a general toxic condition of the animal body caused by long-term health degeneration of ancestors—and in the case of young puppy losses—of parent stock, the only remedy for which is, as in the case of the agricultural testament from which I have just previously quoted, not suppression of the symptoms by use of the highly dangerous sulphonamide drugs, but by getting down to root causes, and as to which there is no call again to repeat myself—sufficient to state now merely the two words, *bad rearing*.

There can be no denying, however, that there are, in dogs, diseases of the reproductive organs very similar to the venereal diseases of the human body. Now many eminent doctors hold the rightful theory that such disease is mostly of a mucous or catarrhal nature, and is in part a self-cleansing attempt of the body. It must be agreed, however, that there is some degree of contagion, the disease being passed from stud dog to bitch during mating. (But consider the large number of bitches which do have venereal infection—metritis is such an infection—entirely independent of any sexual intercourse whatsoever; maiden bitches quite commonly develop this disease.) Though even in contact with active disease, good health is an absolute safeguard; no stud dog could infect a really healthy bitch, and vice versa, for the bacteria must find unhealthy tissues on which to feed and multiply, and would very soon perish in the healthy alkaline tissues of the reproductive organs of a well-reared dog or bitch. Breeders, therefore, should not be too ready to blame infection on other people's stud dogs or bitches: let them look to the health of their own stock first, and remember that true health provides immunity to all disease, including worm infestation.

Professor A. Ehret, brilliant German professor of human medicine, son of a veterinary surgeon, author of many far-seeing

Ailments and Their Treatments

English-written books on dietetics (on which he was an acknowledged great authority), has written words of much wisdom concerning venereal disease, which writings are completely in agreement with my own theories concerning such disease in human and veterinary medicine.

To quote from his writings: 'There is no principal difference between any one kind of disease or another. In the case of venereal disease there is an exception, but only so far as symptoms of syphilis are concerned. Venereal disease can be healed by diet and fasting easily, for the simple reason that the patient is generally young in years. The cure becomes more difficult if drugs have been used. This unfortunately has happened in almost every case. The so-called characteristic symptoms of any kind of syphilitic disease are due to drugs of one or several kinds. . . . Gonorrhoea. Nothing is easier to heal than this "cold" or "catarrh" of the sex organs, if untouched by drugs. Doctors must admit that the condition may exist without actual sexual intercourse, and therefore the germ can hardly be blamed. Gonorrhoea is simply an elimination through the natural elimination organ. If drug injections are used for any continual length of time, the mucus and pus are thrown back into the prostatic gland, bladder, etc. In the case of the female the entire womb, uterus, becomes inflamed, producing all kinds of typical women's diseases . . . Roseola or rose rash. A syphilitical eczema is due to the saltpetre-acid, silver-oxide injections. This is also the cause if gonorrhoea enters the bone. All are called syphilitic symptoms. Mercury is to blame for the hard chancre, secondary and tertiary syphilis.'

Mr. James C. Thompson, principal of the Edinburgh School of Natural Therapeutics, has drawn attention to the findings of Dr. Hermann, of Vienna (whose findings, in the same way as Professor Ehret's, help to undo much of the mischievous work of such popular scientists as Koch and Ehrlich). Dr. Hermann found, in connection with the harmful chemical drug treatment of venereal diseases, that during thirty years' work on venereal disease he had treated over sixty thousand patients, and among the thousands of syphilitic cases which he treated without use of the chemical—mercury—not one case developed symptoms of constitutional syphilis; whereas in the cases of so-called constitutional syphilis which came to the Hospital Weiden in Vienna, Dr. Hermann found that all had histories of the mercurial treatment, and he

Ailments and Their Treatments

pointed out that workers in the Idria mercury mines, who had never had syphilis infection, developed symptoms identical with those of cases of so-called secondary or tertiary syphilis. He therefore stated, with authority, that the symptoms commonly diagnosed as constitutional syphilis were in fact due to the effects of mercury in the human body.

The foregoing is all of interest because it does well illustrate the harm done by the suppression of symptoms with chemicals. At present, the veterinary profession are mostly treating b.h.s. in dogs with either sulphonamide drugs or vaccines. If anything, the latter are less harmful than the former, for the damage done to various organs of the body by sulphonamides—especially to the kidneys and to the nervous system—is so difficult to remedy. Even supposedly 'simple' chemical tonic powders, in such wide use among pet dogs, may have a drug-accumulative effect in the canine body which is the cause of early senility, rheumatism, eye ailments, and many other abnormal body developments. The one and only cure for b.h.s. is a thorough internal cleansing of the body through fasting, use of harmless herbal medicines, and a corrective raw-foods diet, all of which will remove the basic causes of the state of disease; cure usually takes from two to three months. But stock must not be bred from until six months following the satisfactory termination of the internal cleansing treatment. I have not yet heard of a single instance where cleansed stock have failed to breed normally.

Two cases deserve special mention here. The first concerns a cocker spaniel bitch owned by Mrs. Jordan, of Elmwood Road, Upton Lea, Slough. The ill-health symptom in this bitch was prolonged severe *bowel* trouble, and yet a leading veterinary authority on streptococcal disease had diagnosed the trouble as b.h.s. infection and had ordered a long course of injections. An old bitch which had always proved sterile was pronounced a 'germ carrier of b.h.s. infections' and also had to suffer a long course of injections. The injections gave no improvement, and Mrs. Jordan, reading in a canine journal of a red setter cured of a bowel condition similar to her bitch's by a course of my herbal treatment, wrote to me. On my instruction she immediately left off the b.h.s. injections and treated the bitch on the method described in this Streptococcal section. The bitch had been under injection treatment for over four months; the herbal treatment healed the bowels

165

in five days! Neither dog received another injection. The cocker bitch remained in good health once the bowel trouble had been overcome. One year later the bitch was bred from and had an easy whelping of seven puppies, all of which were reared. To quote Mrs. Jordan: 'All the pups grew up very fit and strong, I had no trouble whatever. You will remember the dam was a b.h.s. victim.'

The second case, of very special interest for the research work, was an Alsatian bitch owned by the Templefield Kennels, of Mrs. J. Parr, Buxton. A bitch which for several years had been carefully reared on natural-rearing methods, by Mrs. J. Ixer, had been kennelled with other so-called b.h.s. cases. The owner of the stud dog to which the bitch was to be sent asked that the bitch should be tested for b.h.s. She was tested and found to be 'positive'. The tests were submitted to 'expert specialist' advice, and treatment with a course of specially prepared vaccine was prescribed for the bitch, together with similar treatment for all animals with which the bitch had been in contact. Ignoring such advice, Mrs. Parr wrote me, and, with Mrs. Ixer's consent, it was decided to make a 'test case' of this Alsatian bitch. She was therefore mated to Mrs. Parr's own stud dog, and has since whelped a perfectly normal litter, all of which were weaned easily. The puppies proved to be very healthy and exceptionally forward (always the case when the bitch has been given strictct pre-natal care with regard to diet and exercise). There was no doubt at all that the litter would grow up into healthy adulthood in the same way as so many condemned litters from other b.h.s.-diagnosed stock.[1] It must in fairness be stated that the veterinary profession has itself issued the statement in the *Veterinary Record*—and quoted in *Our Dogs*—that 'B.H.S. can be isolated from the vaginas of most healthy bitches, so that its presence in swabs taken does not necessarily signify that it was the cause of the trouble' (abortion, death of suckling puppies, and sterility in the bitch).

The lesson learned from both of the above examples is—that if the owners of the bitches concerned had not taken matters into their own hands, the bitches would no doubt have suffered long-term vaccine treatment, together with the destructive effect on the nerves caused by such form of treatment.

[1] A bitch puppy from this litter was a First Prize winner at the great show of the Alsatian League, February 1946. The stud dog was awarded **Best Dog in Show**.

Ailments and Their Treatments

In an effective article in *Our Dogs*, January 1954, entitled 'The Worm in the Apple—Infertility', Vivienne Ferguson writes as follows: 'In addition to the normal hazards of keeping pedigree livestock of all kinds, another problem is causing worry to breeders. I refer to the problem of Fertility and the early death or even still-birth of the progeny.

'This is a problem which has always existed, but there seems little doubt that it is steadily increasing and may eventually threaten the actual existence of certain strains or even certain breeds of dogs, as has already happened in different fields of animal husbandry. . . .

'*Not Always the Parents*. To show that not all cases of high mortality are due to faulty stock, I will quote an instance with my own dogs which occurred about fourteen years ago, and which was doubtless due to bad management on my part.

'My bitches seldom missed, but though the puppies were born alive, seldom more than one survived to the end of the week. . . . Despite skilled veterinary attention, blood tests, swabs, injections of various kinds and everything from the sulphonamides to autogenous vaccines, the only benefit was to my veterinary surgeon's pocket.

'In despair, after resting the buildings, and thoroughly disinfecting everything, I drastically fasted my rather battered dogs (using the herbal cleansing method of Juliette de Baïracli-Levy) and switched completely to natural feeding and management. One year later, my dogs, looking the picture of health, were rearing every puppy and there has been no further trouble.'

Treatment. All b.h.s. conditions, as in the case of venereal diseases of the human body, are infections of the mucous membranes, and are therefore largely catarrhal. Internal cleansing, together with most strict supervision of kennelling conditions, is the proved cure. The advice on distemper treatment, i.e. internal-cleansing fasting treatment, as given in this book, must be strictly followed. But whereas distemper treatment is usually of merely three weeks' duration, b.h.s. treatment requires as a rule three *months* following the short fast to get the reproductive system really cleansed and restored to normal health. Reproduction is the most strenuous function of the living body, and if the body is unhealthy or drug saturated, then all manner of abnormalities can be expected in either the parents or the offspring of unhealthy

Ailments and Their Treatments

stock. How breeders can deliberately mate unhealthy stock just for the sake of getting puppies to sell I really cannot understand; the mean things that people will do for money-gain is an astonishing factor in human nature. One day it will be appreciated that the only true wealth is good health of both body and mind: 80 per cent of present-day domestic animals are unhealthy. To sum up: internal treatment is purely cleansing, followed by body building on a healthful raw diet; also a six months' period of rest from all reproduction activity for both stud dogs and bitches.

Raspberry leaf, on account of its tonic effect on the organs of reproduction, can be used with great advantage for both dogs and bitches. Make a standard brew, and give a dose of the brew morning and evening for approximately three to six weeks. Average dose is two tablespoonfuls morning and evening. For external cleansing of the reproductive organs, any of the aromatic herbs made into an infusion by the standard method are helpful—*sage*, *thyme*, *rosemary* or *blackberry* leaf infusion as used so successfully in eczema treatment can be used. Leaf-extract tablets (natural chlorophyll) are more effective than the garlic for the prolonged treatment which follows the ten to eighteen days of internal cleansing treatment.

Dog owners need have no fear concerning streptococcal infection. It is a disease confined solely to unhealthy, ill-reared stock, and is a natural result of overcrowded conditions. No well-reared animals can be affected. Keep small numbers of dogs only; feed them on the highest quality raw foods, give them the abundant free running exercise which their nature craves, let them grow up from puppyhood on clean grassland, and b.h.s. disease, together with all disease, will pass such dogs by. In years of Afghan hound puppy rearing I have never given disease a thought among my own dogs, and stock of my 'Turkuman' prefix has been among the most eagerly sought stock in England, and has been chosen as foundation stock by leading kennels in England and America; the extraordinary good health of my N.R. stock was one of their chief attractions. Other breeders of other breeds, concentrating on the rearing of healthy stock, have had the same experience and have found the same great demand for their stock. Health must be valued as highly as any show points; it is, indeed, of higher value —it being indispensable to the happiness of the dog and its survival.

Ailments and Their Treatments

STUTTGART DISEASE. This is a contagious disease which takes a rapid course, and if not treated immediately, can prove fatal. Symptoms are incessant vomiting and great thirst; the tongue often turns black. There is dysentery, sometimes with bleeding.

Treatment. Treat as for distemper (see Distemper). Give an extra-strong dose of herbal antiseptic tablets or infusion of antiseptic herbs such as *garlic*. Treat the vomiting with *gentian* (see Sickness).

THINNESS. (See treatments under Appetite and also Nervousness.) Observe the case carefully for worms; if detected, then treat. It should be pointed out that most people like the domestic dog over-fat. The dog in natural health is, like the wolf, a lean, swift animal.

Treatment. Increase rations of whole-grain cereal foods, feed some slices of buttered wholewheat bread daily. Give minced *celery* mixed into the meat, especially the leaves. *Fenugreek* seed is a great fattener and has been used through the ages to fatten horses. Soak the seed for twenty-four hours, using warm water. When soft mix with the usual cereal meal. Also raisins can be fed in the morning, like pills into the mouth. Several dessertspoons early morning.

THYROID. This is a glandular ailment. Treat as for obesity (see Obesity). Give especially all the iodine-rich herbs and foods: *seaweed*, *garlic*, egg yolks, raw.

TICK FEVER. This is more prevalent in very hot climates. The dog develops a fever and loses weight with alarming speed. Death can result.

Treatment. This has been very successful and my herbal treatment with *garlic* is well known in South Africa. Treat on distemper lines (see Distemper) with fasting and saturating the blood-stream with garlic, *eucalyptus* (a brew of the leaves), and other antiseptic herbs. For external protection against ticks, dust the dog regularly with herbal insecticide powder. During the tick season give sea salt on the food and increase the daily ration of *seaweed*.

TUMOURS. (See Breast Tumours.)

WARTS. Warts are usually a sign of glandular derangement, although they can sometimes be Nature's action of isolating body toxins beneath the skin surface. Do not use surgery.

Treatment. The best treatment is internal, through diet. Feed plenty of raw minced *dandelion* leaves; also crushed boiled *broad*

169

beans, given with the meat feed, are helpful. The best medicine, apart from diet, is seaweed powder, because of its high natural iodine content. For external treatment, the gypsies place great faith in the juice from stems or roots of *dandelion* or *greater celandine.* Squeeze out the milky-looking juice, touch the warts with the juice and allow to dry on. Apply the juice three times daily. The stalks of unripe green *figs* yield an excellent milky caustic juice for applying to warts. Also the white milky juice yielded when the skin of unripe *papaya* fruit is punctured.

WORMS. This is one of the most important subjects in this book, because more puppies and adults are actually killed or made permanent invalids through the mischievous and very common practice of worming with strong and irritant chemical drugs and purges than would ever die from the presence of worms themselves, or from any of the other common ailments of puppyhood.

I must begin by saying that, in spite of the advance in science, the subject of helminthology continues to remain 'wrapt in mystery'; what a far greater service scientists would render, both to humanity and the animal races, if they would devote more time to the study of parasitical worms, instead of spending all of their time and energies on research connected with Pasteur's discredited germ theory—that is, discredited by most thinking people. At present we know little beyond the fact that there are two types of worms which infect dogs: round worms and tapeworms, both types of which are divided into several varieties. And, further, that the ova of the worms enter the dog through the mouth, doing so from many sources: from infested ground (worm ova can lie dormant for years in soil); from stagnant, or even running, water, to which other dogs or sheep or vermin—such as rabbits or rats—have access; from the milk of an infected bitch—in the case of puppies; from fleas which are carriers of a species of tapeworm; from worm-infected intestines of rabbits, cattle, or poultry; or from the flesh of such animals where the worm is then present in an encysted state.

It should be appreciated from the above details that if such a minute creature as a flea can be a host for a tapeworm, the larvae of the blowfly and other meat- and carrion-eating flies may well be worm-carriers also, as may be the flies themselves. Wild birds are often infected with worms, and domestic poultry very commonly are. The droppings of birds very soon dry into a dust-like con-

Ailments and Their Treatments

sistency and spread over grassland, thus forming a very likely source of worms in dogs and other livestock. All this merely proves that it is almost *impossible* to prevent a dog, especially a puppy, from absorbing worms into its system from one source or another during its lifetime. But what is possible is—the prevention of the worm eggs from ever developing into the adult worm, or, having developed, from breeding to an extent which would bring about worm infestation. The presence of a few round worms in the adult dog or puppy is no cause for alarm; as I shall prove later in this section on worms, their presence might even do good. It is only infestation which is harmful: and the only and certain way to prevent that state being reached is to keep the entire internal system of the dog, including the blood-stream, in a clean, healthy condition by means of careful and correct rearing, which includes hygienic kennelling and regular fasting. The presence of tapeworm is more serious than round worms, owing to the fact that the head of the tapeworm is armed with many hooks which attach themselves to the mucous membranes in various parts of the body, and these hooks may exert a harmful tearing action; while, further, the tapeworm generally excretes as waste matter a fluid which is an irritant to the dog's system, especially to the nerves and brain. But unlike the round worms, a tapeworm can rarely establish itself in a clean digestive tract, for it relies upon mucus deposits beneath which to shelter itself: the very presence of a tapeworm denotes unclean internal conditions. Though I must add that although the presence of a tapeworm in the body is known to cause some harm, it may also, as in the case of the round worm—which I shall give later—do a certain amount of good by absorbing a quantity of the sour food deposits and other toxic accumulations found in an unhealthy digestive tract.

I need to classify here more definitely the two types of canine worms, although there is no space in this book for any detailed descriptions—for such, a veterinary medicine textbook should be referred to. I will deal firstly with round worms, of which there are two distinct classes, although this fact is seldom realized by dog breeders. The type most generally found is the *Ascarides lumbricoides*, which again can be subdivided into several distinct species, but all of which usually inhabit the small intestine, although when a state of infestation is reached they may leave their usual habitat and crawl into the stomach, or enter the bile duct (causing

171

jaundice), or even invade the lungs, the nostrils, or the eyes. The other type is the *Ascarides vermiculares*, which inhabits the rectum and large intestines; and, in bitches, may spread into the vagina. The tapeworm family are classified under the name of *Taenia*, of which there are many varieties, but which cannot be clearly divided into distinct classes as in the case of the round worms.

(1) Round worms: Ascarides lumbricoides. The modern veterinary treatment of rapid blasting out of the worms, with no regard to the sensitive structure of the digestive system, is not only useless but extremely harmful. For the health of the entire body is greatly dependent upon a sound digestive tract, and once the health of that important part of the body is destroyed by irritant vermicides —nearly all drug vermicides depend upon irritant properties for the removal of the worms—not only does the entire health of the puppy, or adult, suffer, but the weakened intestines become very suitable breeding-grounds for any further worms which may invade the body, and which will certainly then reproduce themselves in yet greater numbers in the weakened intestines or stomach which can now offer little resistance to the invading parasite. If the second crop of worms are removed by the same method, which method may even be repeated a third time, the resultant state of the dog's health can well be imagined. It is at such times that a condition of worm infestation is subsequently established, followed in many cases by the painful death of the puppy or even of the adult. It is also under such conditions that the disease-resisting powers of the dog become so lowered that one of the infectious diseases, frequently distemper or streptococcal infection, develops, and when the dog is seriously worm-infested its chances of recovery are then very slight, for the internal healing powers natural to every living creature will in such circumstances be but very feeble indeed. It can therefore be appreciated that treatment with potent drug vermifuges is worse than useless—it is killing; and such treatments are today killing off hundreds of puppies or, if not killing, permanently destroying the sound health which is the true birthright of all living things. In the treatment of all types of worms the best treatment is preventive; in the case of puppies, commence this treatment before birth by disinfecting the blood-stream of the dam (in which the worm eggs travel), and later the milk flow by the use of garlic; then the correct rearing of the puppies on natural rearing methods, in order to ensure a strong, vigorous stomach

Ailments and Their Treatments

and intestines, and healthy, pure blood-stream, the possession of which would never permit a state of worm infestation, but which would ensure the natural expulsion in the daily evacuation of faeces of any worms which have entered in egg form via the mouth and developed. But in the very usual case of a person purchasing worm-infested dogs, herbal treatment supplies safe and effective removal of the parasites.

Treatment. Worm Infestation. Commence with a water-only fast of one day for a young puppy, two days for a puppy over six months or for an adult. Young puppies can have a little honey added, approximately one teaspoon per water dish, for an average-size puppy. On the night of the fast give a strong dose of *castor* oil; one dessertspoon for an average-size puppy under six months, less for a puppy under three months. A much increased dose for older dogs, i.e. one and one-half tablespoons for an adult cocker-size dog, two tablespoons for an adult greyhound-type dog.

The following day, commence the treatment proper. A strong dose of herbal tablets, approximately six to eight, three-grain tablets, containing such herbs as *garlic, rue, eucalyptus,* etc., or other herbal worming tablets. Thirty minutes later give a further laxative dose of castor oil, the same quantities as above. Thirty minutes later give a warm, laxative feed of milk thickened with tree-barks flour and honey, some flaked oats added. The meal should be semi-liquid. If the dog's stomach is very upset from prolonged worms, it may vomit this meal, which should then be newly prepared and given again after the lapse of thirty minutes. The tree-barks flour acts as a soothing jelly which passes through the intestines, removing worms and their eggs.

Meals following wormings should be small, a cupful of liquid food for a six-month-old cocker, for example. Keep the dog on this fluid diet of three small meals of milk and honey, tree barks and cereal, for at least three days. A little whole-maize flour can be added, raw.

When the stomach and intestines are ulcerated from worm infestation, it is essential to rest them for a short period on a light diet of semi-fluid foods. Throughout the fluid diet give the early morning dose of herbal tablets, but cut the dose by half, i.e. if six tablets were given for the worming, then reduce to three tablets for the morning continuation dose. Also, each night it is advisable to give a laxative of a mild and cleansing kind, such as *senna* pods.

173

Ailments and Their Treatments

An average puppy dose of one large pod soaked in one tablespoon of cold water, with a pinch of ground *ginger* added to prevent griping. Senna dose for an adult greyhound would be four large senna pods soaked in the same way, using two tablespoons of cold water, with ginger added.

Now return the case to a normal diet, slowly introducing the N.R. raw-foods diet meals (see diet charts for puppies and adults, Chapter 1). Once solid foods have been restored to the diet, cease the night-time laxative. But add to the daily diet for some time worm-removing aids, such as grated raw *coconut*, grated raw *carrot*, ground *pumpkin* seeds (raw), cut seeds, raw, of *nasturtium* and of *papaya*, whole *grape* seeds, whole *melon* pips, finely chopped raw *garlic*. Do not aim to add all of these; one or two of these items would be beneficial. An average amount for a puppy of average breed would be one teaspoon of any one of them, or one dessertspoon for a cocker-size adult, given twice daily.

Also give two or three herbal tablets daily, average-size dog, for approximately eighteen days.

In the case of puppies reinfecting themselves from sour ground or ova-impregnated kennel floors or dirty yards, the worm treatment should be repeated for several days each month. Treatment is entirely harmless and is indeed internally tonic and cleansing, leaving the dog in better health than before treatment.

In all worm treatments it is a good thing to prepare the dog by starving the worm for several days before actual treatment is given. That is, do not feed foods known to be preferred by worms: fats, sugars, eggs, milk. Feed mainly flaked oats, skimmed and watered milk to soften the oats, and lightly boiled fish in place of raw or cooked meat.

Timing of worm treatment. The ancient people always recognized the fact that worms are greatly influenced by the moon. Worms become more active and commence breeding when the moon is waxing, they are less buried then in the tissues of their prey, therefore that is the correct time to plan worm treatment, when the moon is waxing, and then carrying out the actual deep cleansing with castor oil and herbal tablets *just before* full moon. I have well proved this theory in the worming treatment of dogs, goats, cows, and horses; the ancient belief, typical of many ancient things in medicine, was founded on intelligent observation by primitive man, taught by his own experience instead of from medical text-books.

174

Ailments and Their Treatments

Alternative worm treatments. When the usual worming herbs as already given are not available, others may be used. *Mustard seed:* The seed is ground into a fine powder and given as worm seed. Average dose is one dessertspoon given in two tablespoons warmed skimmed milk. Or a mustard-plant infusion can be made by the usual strong infusion (see Chapter 5), using both leaves and flowers of the wild mustard plant. Follow the mustard with castor oil and the usual worming treatment as described above. Or *walnut* leaves: make a strong infusion, two tablespoons of the infusion being given during fasting, followed by castor oil.

(2) Round worms: Ascarides vermiculares. Enema treatments are necessary in addition to the above internal treatment as for round worms. A tepid solution of *tobacco* infused by the standard method. Or two tablespoons of the finely shredded leaves of the same plant, same infusion. In this enema treatment at least a half pint of infusion, for an average-size dog, should be injected into the anus. Then, after the enema has been expelled, the anus should be bathed with an infusion of *lavender* or *rosemary* plant. As *Ascarides vermiculares* will also infect the vagina of female animals, vaginal treatments with rosemary or lavender infusion should be used.

(3) Hook worm: Ancylostoma caninum. When present to the extent of infestation, these cause a disease known as ancylostomiasis, a form of severe anaemia due to the blood-sucking action peculiar to hook worms, which can even attack the muscles.

Treatment. Same as for round worms, (see foregoing). Treat also for Anaemia, see this chapter.

(4) Tapeworm. This is a far more difficult parasite to expel than the round worm, for once it has established itself in the dog's body it is armed by Nature against attempts to dislodge it, the head of the tapeworm being provided with a sucker, and also a circle of hooks with which it digs itself into the mucous membrane; while it further protects itself by burying its body beneath mucus and other deposits which are invariably found in an unclean digestive tract. It is said in the East, by the Arabs, that only 'a foul body breeds loathsome worms', and it is further claimed that it is the partaking of cooked food—which is dead food—which causes worms. This opinion is, of course, contrary to the scientific fact that only by cooking flesh foods can the encysted forms of tape and other worms be destroyed. However, cooked food is 'dead'

Ailments and Their Treatments

food, and means a general loss of health, and I myself have carefully proved that when cooked meat is regularly fed to dogs in place of the natural raw meat, worm trouble, especially tapeworm, is very frequent; no doubt this is due to the toxic accumulations from cooked foods which provide good breeding-ground for worms, and thus encourage their presence. The harm that tapeworms cause in the body has been described earlier in this worm section.

Treatment. In tapeworm it is necessary to expel the head, for as long as the head remains the worm will continue to produce segments, each segment being itself a complete worm capable of developing into an independent worm. Treatment is primarily internal cleansing, and the complete treatment for round worm (*Ascarides lumbricoides*) should be followed. *Garlic* is a specific for tapeworm and has given excellent results, especially when combined with other antiseptic herbs. Dosage must be very strong, following the usual castor oil and fasting treatment (see Round worms). An average dose for the spaniel-size dog would be six three-grain tablets. Alternative herbal treatments are oil of *male fern*, taken from the roots of the fern *Aspidium filix mas.*; this oil can be purchased from many chemists as it is still in use for human tapeworm treatment. Ask the pharmacist to prescribe dosage according to weight of dog; a common dose is one-half ounce male fern oil mixed with one-half ounce corn oil. One teaspoon of the mixture is then given after the usual twenty-four hours' fasting, with castor oil before and after. Also in use are *areca* and *pomegranate*. *Areca* nuts are from a species of palm tree and were once in very popular use. They are rather strong medicine for use on the modern dog with its weakened intestinal tracts resulting from unnatural rearing. But they are of service for the big breeds when herbal tablets are not obtainable. The nut contains an active ingredient, *arecoline*, which causes worms to loosen their grip on the tissue of their host. The nut should be freshly rubbed on a nutmeg grater for immediate use after the standard fasting castor-oil preparation, for the nut loses its value speedily after exposure to air. The required amount of powder is taken and mixed into a mass with thick honey and a little flour, using the tip of a dry knife.

Divide this bolus into several pills and press down the dog's throat. An average dose is one-half teaspoon of the nut (before mixing) for fully matured puppies or adults of an average breed.

Ailments and Their Treatments

Do not use areca for young puppies, in-whelp bitches, or toy breeds.

Pomegranate possesses an active worm-expellent ingredient, *pelletierine*, present in the rind of the fruit and more strongly in the bark of the root. The rind or bark, purchased from a herbalist, should be freshly powdered and prepared as described for male fern root, but no senna need be added. Pomegranate should also be used in conjunction with the fasting castor-oil treatment.

Charcoal, given in tablet form, is a useful addition to all worm treatments, when normal feeding is restored. Charcoal absorbs impurities from the internal organs, but it should not be used for longer than one month, with long intervals in between use, as it is apt to absorb too much from the body, including the good with the bad.

WOUNDS. (See Bleeding of Wounds.)

Final Note. If your dog should become ill, and as a dog owner you have no experience of sickness, do send to a veterinary surgeon for his diagnosis, telling him firmly that you wish to treat the ailment with herbs. I am sure that he will prove to be both helpful and interested. Please do not write to me for personal advice. I have written my herbal book with its carefully worked-out treatments for readers to carry out the treatments for themselves. I am away on my travels, and letters requesting veterinary help usually reach me months late, the dog probably having fully recovered by then; many do not reach me at all. I corresponded in former days when I was not travelling and could provide no detailed treatments in book form. Now I have this book which is fully able to answer all queries on treatments of diseases in dogs.

Part Three

7

The Failure of Disease Prevention
through Vaccination

Vaccination, although originated by the English country doctor Edward Jenner, has been based largely on the germ theory of the French chemist, Louis Pasteur.

Pasteur was not able to keep his own body in good health and he suffered from paralysis of the mouth in his later years; he also lost, from disease, members of his own family. I have always believed in 'Healer, heal thyself first!' Then you have the authority to teach others how to heal themselves. If I had not been able to keep my own Afghan hounds, goats, and horses in good health, I would never have possessed my absolute faith in herbal medicine and nature rearing, and would not have written my herbal books, or this present book, which brings right up to date my herbal work and gives over one hundred new and proven herbal treatments.

I have also watched my beliefs concerning the inability of vaccination to prevent canine disease come to be sadly, and overwhelmingly, proved correct. Disease rate among modern dogs has not been lowered by mass vaccination; it is greatly on the increase. Vaccination has produced numerous carriers of virulent diseases, or the treated dogs themselves, often given triple vaccinations nowadays, often develop all three of these very ailments—and die a speedy death.

The plague diseases of former days have not been controlled by vaccination; they owe their decline to those few benefits which man has derived from modern medicine: from improved sanitation and housing.

As I write this, I have before me a copy of the newspaper, *San*

The Failure of Disease Prevention

Diego Union, sponsoring one of those frequent articles trying to encourage mankind to accept more completely the practice of vaccination. Now vaccination is an exceedingly profitable business, both to the manufacturers of vaccine and to the distributors of these unnatural products: it will decline very slowly in popular esteem, if it is ever allowed to die at all. Press advertising determinedly keeps vaccination to the fore. The San Diego newspaper article was meant to be in favour of vaccination and was recommending 'booster shots' for human use. The advice is given that several dozen vaccinations should be taken during a human lifetime, vaccinating many times against polio, smallpox, tetanus. The concluding advice is then given: 'Does "being vaccinated" mean that you are forever safe from a disease? No! No! . . . stamping out epidemics does not mean that all the people who have been vaccinated are totally immune to the disease. You do need boosters.'

That vaccination has an insidious effect on general canine health has been noted by observant dog breeders. It is one of the causes of chronic skin disease, especially of the mange form. Also, greyhound owners have noted that vaccination has an adverse effect on the speed of their racing dogs. Mr. James Baldwin, the well-known greyhound authority and breeder also of German shepherd dogs, wrote in *Dog World* concerning an anti-distemper vaccination movement among Irish and English greyhound breeders, resulting from the adverse effects on the natural speed of their dogs, and in support of this he published a long statement from a greyhound man, whom he described as being 'one of England's most successful and experienced greyhound trainers that there has ever been'—giving his proof that vaccination made swift dogs slow.

In Switzerland many leading veterinary surgeons oppose distemper vaccination, declaring that it gives little protection and often undermines health; and in modern Israel there is very little canine vaccine used, popular veterinary opinion being that it is useless and often gives the disease in a severe form to young stock who otherwise might never have the disease. I do not know of one dog in Tiberias, Israel (where I now live fairly permanently) which has had canine distemper vaccination.

Personally I have no use for vaccinations whatsoever, and although during my travels my young children and my dogs who accompany me are exposed to numerous new contagious ailments,

182

The Failure of Disease Prevention

the only protection which I desire for them is the all-round protection of good health resulting from careful daily diet of good, whole, natural foods, mostly eaten raw—as Nature intended for man and animals—also the use of disinfectant herbs.

In his writings, Dr. Franz Hartmann, M.D., a great Theosophist, warns against vaccination. 'It would be interesting to find out how many chronic diseases and life-long evils are caused by vaccination.'

Dr. Douglas Latto, M.D., Ch.B., D.R.C.O.G., informs in his pamphlet, *The Fruits of Vivisection*: 'It is recognized that diphtheria immunization increases one's chance of getting infantile paralysis, and during an outbreak of infantile paralysis (*anterior poliomyelitis*) it is customary now to stop diphtheria immunization.'

The famed homeopathic doctor, Dorothy Shepherd, M.D., condemning vaccination, has written: 'The more I follow up clinical histories, the more I am inclined to agree with opponents of vaccination, that vaccination instead of being a blessing has proved to be a wolf in sheep's clothing, and has produced more misery, more ill health, in its wake than almost any other method of treatment.'

There follow the opinions of two eminent doctors concerning distemper immunization; first, I quote Dr. J. E. R. McDonagh, F.R.C.S., the bacteriologist, in *The Nature of Disease*, Volume I, pp. 75–6: 'Immunization with an attenuated virus cannot prevent distemper. The author has treated many dogs, which have developed distemper despite two or three injections of the preventative agent. . . . He is of the opinion that fits, chorea, hysteria, etc., in dogs, have become more frequent since the use of Distemper Vaccine. Successful prevention will never be achieved by inoculation.'

And the other doctor, Dr. W. J. Murphy—who 'before becoming a physician' was 'a graduated veterinarian' for fifteen years—expresses the opinion (which is absolutely my own opinion, and is now also the opinion of large numbers of dog breeders and owners): 'No serum nor virus for distemper is necessary nor can it accomplish any good for an ailment that has a natural tendency to get well of itself.'

Then famous people in the world of dogs have also given valuable and experienced opinion on this unnatural vaccination method of attempting to prevent diseases which come to domestic animals through man's unnatural rearing methods, which have shown no improvement or reform, but yearly increase in their unnaturalness.

Herewith I quote six opinions selected from the thirty which I published in the English first edition of my canine herbal book, which is still available in libraries.

1. LEO C. WILSON, journalist and international judge, writes in *Our Dogs*, England (1955). 'People should not place too much faith in any form of inoculation against virus diseases since none yet discovered guarantees immunity. This is not to say that such inoculations are worthless but there is great danger that if people think that the inoculations do give positive immunity they are likely to take risks with their dogs which they would otherwise avoid and herein lies the pitfall.'

2. CLIFFORD HUBBARD, international canine authority and author, contributor to *Our Dogs, Dog World, The Field*, etc. Author of *Dogs in Britain, The Observer Book of Dogs*, etc. 'I have just read for the third time your book on *The Cure of Canine Distemper*. I am completely in agreement with you on your views *against* the so-called immunization of dogs against distemper by the injection of various potent vaccines the exact micro-organism content of which must always remain unknown, and I admire your courage and sincerity of purpose in denouncing the orthodox treatment.'

3. A. W. SALZMANN, chemist, Beundenfeldstrasse, 32, Bern, Switzerland: 'Dr. Hermann Reitzer, of Vienna, has mentioned your veterinary book that distemper in dogs can be cured. Last year I lost three very wonderful Gordon Setters, and I do not need to tell you how eagerly I am looking forward to a cure. I am dealing already in serums, especially made to prevent distemper, but I am by now *convinced that no serum will help*. My dogs died of distemper in spite of vaccination.'

4. M. MARCHANT, Greyhound breeder, 142 Tickford Street, Newport Pagnell, Bucks. 'I have great confidence in your distemper writings, especially as my mother who manages one of the Union Greyhound stud farms in South Africa, writes me that 50 valuable dogs were lost last year at their farm, all were inoculated. I cannot imagine why dog breeders should remain blind to the dangers of this orthodox treatment. I myself have had a favourite dog ruined by such treatment, and in a recent distemper epidemic two dogs survived out of 20.'

The Failure of Disease Prevention

5. G. Messenger, 10 Hunter's Road, Hockley, Birmingham. 'I am in full agreement with all you state as to inoculation for distemper. The remedy is worse than the disease. You could not give me a dog if I knew it had been inoculated. The dog world owes you much for your exposure of this so-called cure; also for your real cure and remedies. I am no novice, having been breeding for 47 years, and exhibiting for 37 years.'

6. George Muir, P.O. Box 470, Place d'Armes, Montreal, Canada. 'I have been very interested in your writings in *Our Dogs* on the subject of distemper inoculation and I have seen in the American *Dog World* that you have published a book on the distemper subject. Recently my interest in distemper has become very active, having just lost a very fine St. Bernard female puppy two weeks after having the first of three inoculations under the ————method.

'All those with whom I have since discussed the subject and who were in favour of inoculation, all maintained that the injections could not in any way affect the dog. Then they proceeded to contradict themselves by adding one or more of the following reservations: Don't inoculate during teething. Don't inoculate unless the dog is in perfect condition. Don't inoculate during Fall season (in Canada) as weather is so changeable. After inoculation, only exercise the dog but little for 7 days. After inoculation, don't allow contact with other dogs—7 days. After inoculation, make sure that the dog is in no way subjected to draughts, etc.

'Now why should all these reservations be made if the inoculation has no effect on the victim? The common-sense deduction to be made is in my opinion—inoculation reduces the natural disease resistance of a healthy animal—even although administered by experts; and who, in his own opinion at least, is not an expert?'

I quote the following, without comment, from the American *Dog World*:

'I had five German shepherd puppies inoculated against distemper. The veterinarian recommended and used the — method. With each puppy we received an inoculation certificate. At a later date another kennel purchased these puppies along with an older male; the puppies were in good health. After they had had them for about one month, they sold three to individual buyers, and kept two of them and the older male for themselves. All of the six months puppies developed distemper and died, the ten months

185

The Failure of Disease Prevention

male, who was not inoculated and was kennelled in the same building, never acquired this disease. Are we in any way obligated to this kennel for the deaths of these puppies? . . . And *what is your opinion concerning the —— method?'*

(The italicizing of this last line is mine.—J. de B.-L.)

And here is a further quote from a letter which reached me recently and was not meant to criticize vaccination:

From Mrs. A. M. Dryland, Bowenhurst, Church Crookham, Hants: 'I have a Labrador bitch, and she was inoculated with —— against distemper and hard pad, as her breeder was very insistent on this. However, when we came here my bitch got distemper, and the *vet gave her an injection which he said would clear it up quickly and was the one used when a dog had been inoculated and had developed distemper.'*

(The italics in this quote are again mine.—J. de B.-L.)

All this prompts me to requote from the pro-vaccination article in the *San Diego Union.* 'Does "being vaccinated" mean that you are forever safe from a disease? No! No!'

I was discussing my dislike of inoculation and serum with an important London veterinary surgeon, whose claim was that he inoculated more dogs in a year than perhaps any other veterinary surgeon. He told me that I was being 'foolish, backward, failing to keep pace with modern times', etc., in my attitude towards such 'wonderful discoveries as vaccine and serum'. This veterinary surgeon possessed one dog, one dog only, a Cairn terrier bitch. This one dog belonging to the great supporter of inoculation developed distemper around the time of whelping. Her distemper attack became seriously complicated and not one puppy survived. Yet, during my distemper work, in London, I reared a litter of Afghan puppies in daily contact with the distemper cases that I was treating there. This same veterinary surgeon informed me that it was an act of madness to attempt to rear puppies under such conditions (there were eleven cases of distemper being treated on the premises) and that I would certainly lose every puppy. However, despite the fact that the puppies were seriously handicapped by the mother having been poisoned and the puppies having to be hand-reared, not one puppy developed distemper.

INTENSIVE HERBAL IMMUNIZATION. At such times as one finds that one's dogs have been in contact with other dogs suffering from any contagious disease, it is advisable to treat all immediately

The Failure of Disease Prevention

in the following way. Give them one- or half-a-day fast, with a laxative that same night, and a dose of herbal antiseptic tablets last thing at night. Then daily give them herbal tablets every morning, or pills can be made from minced *garlic*, one drop of *eucalyptus* oil, wholewheat flour, and honey. Roll all the ingredients together and divide into pills—one drop of eucalyptus to every tablespoon of the mixture.

When known to have been in contact with cases of mange skin disease, bathe the dog immediately and rub into the body a lotion made of a standard infusion of *rosemary* or infusion of herbal insecticide, or rub down with a cloth sprinkled with oil of eucalyptus and spirit of camphor.

When taking dogs to shows or public parks, give them a dose of antiseptic herbs immediately before taking them there.

In Swaledale in the English Pennine mountains I had a memorable demonstration of the power of herbs to protect against contagious disease. There, in 1947, I saved around two thousand pedigree Swaledale sheep, condemned as incurable by orthodox medicine, as witnessed by many farmers. There was one field filled with seriously sick sheep suffering from a streptococcal infection causing paralysis and blindness, and the adjoining field filled with well sheep, kept heavily dosed with herbs. Not one of the well sheep became infected from their sick neighbours.

In the late nineteen-sixties, Sr. Alberico Boncompagni Ludovisi of Rome, Italy, treated foot-and-mouth disease with my herbal method. The cases treated recovered, and those immunized with herbal tablets (such as used against canine distemper) did not take the disease.

8

Conclusion

I end my herbal book with the sincere hope that all readers putting into practice these herbal teachings will achieve the same good health which has long been the possession of my own Turkuman Afghan hounds. Success in good health does not come overnight, it may take several generations to undo the bad health which man has been building up in his own life and the life of domestic animals during the past hundred years, when artificiality in medicine, diet, and agriculture began to predominate in the Western world. But success, in time, is sure, because Nature's own laws are unchanging, and Nature does not fail those who obey her simple laws.

As to the value of herbs—why should they possess the wonderful curative properties that I claim for them? The answer can be summed up in one sentence: they, the herbs, are manufactured by Nature, whereas drugs are manufactured by man (in the case of plant drugs, the normal properties of the plant are so destroyed in manufacture that there is usually little of Nature left in them). Now thinking people cannot deny that, try as he may, man cannot improve upon, or even hope ever to equal, the miraculous creations of Nature. Take but one example—the human eye: what an indescribably perfect thing it is, with its self-cleansing and healing mechanism, its remarkable powers of sight. Compare with the living eye the artificial glass eye that is manufactured by man. To that same extent there is in medicine the difference in values from all the products that are manufactured by Nature to those that are man-made. The medicines in herbs are derived from the cosmic forces of sunlight, moonlight, and starlight; from rain and dew and the minerals of the earth's soil layers, as well as the hereditary

188

Conclusion

properties. Any herb can have its medicinal properties analysed to a certain extent; only the cosmic and the hereditary cannot as yet be measured, which is unfortunate, for it is in this 'streaming spirit' of the herb that most of the healing powers are contained. Up to the present time little research has been carried out in connection with the cosmic forces as contained in plants. Two men only have contributed useful knowledge on that subject: Dr. Rudolf Steiner (the originator of biodynamic farming) and Professor Edmond Szekely.

There has always been a great interest in herbs in America, and I feel that this is a result of the ancient Red Indian background. Also the Swiss are very herb-minded, and it is notable that my veterinary herbal books have gone into numerous editions in Switzerland.

One of my greatest inspirations in my herbal work has always been my detestation of vivisection. I am tired of the arguments in favour of this unnatural branch of unnatural chemical medicine, arguments sponsored by the vast sera manufacturing firms. The great and wise reformer of India, Gandhi, speaks clearly concerning this. 'Vivisection in my opinion is the blackest of all black crimes that man is at present committing against God and His fair creatures. We should be able to refuse to live if the price of living be the torture of sentient creatures.'

I want my book to encourage readers to collect their own herbal products fresh from the fields and woods, as I collect them for my own children and my animals: that is the least expensive way, and the quickest, and medicinal herbs are abundant in Great Britain and in the Americas, as the Red Indians and country people once knew.

As for experiments in animal nutrition, I have been informed on several occasions that I must have carried out experiments in order to work out and prove my natural rearing diet method. No! Such testing was never required. Through mere common sense I knew that natural foods, medicines, and hygienic rearing *must* be best. I could never bring myself to divide a litter of puppies and rear one-half on healthy natural foods and watch the others decline on orthodox processed and cooked foods. I therefore reared all puppies by the same natural and healthy method—and as things happened it was other breeders who supplied 'controls' through their own orthodox methods of dog rearing. For instance,

189

Conclusion

I have many times purchased a young Afghan puppy from another breeder's orthodox-reared litter; that puppy, when internally cleansed and then put on to natural rearing, has developed into a strong, great-boned, heavily coated adult, and has kept disease-free; whereas other puppies from the same litter, kept to adult age on the orthodox methods, have developed into weak-boned, poor-coated specimens, and have fallen victims to the common canine ailments, especially worm infestation and the epidemic diseases. Well-known kennels throughout England, throughout the world, indeed, give testimony as to the superior health that natural rearing methods give in comparison to the orthodox, and unnatural, methods.

When I wrote my first article in the journal, *Our Dogs*, some thirty years ago, I warned against the health degeneration which would result if dog breeders persisted in the unnatural. Today we are seeing some of the tragic results of unnatural rearing. Because a cooked and canned food diet dispenses with the need for tearing and chewing, we find whole litters of dogs being born with the normal quota of teeth missing. The pre-molar teeth are not appearing in the jaw. Then through lack of exercise there is the terrible affliction of hip-dysplasia. This means ultimate lameness. None of these abnormalities are found in the wild carnivores, relatives of the dog, such as wolf and jackal. Man's rearing has afflicted such upon the dog, and worse will follow unless immediate reforms are carried out.

The best preventive medicine remains true to the teachings of the ancient Greek doctor Hippocrates, who is considered to this day 'the father of all medicine'. One of Hippocrates's most famous rulings is: 'Let food be your medicine, and let medicine be your food.' And it is said of Hippocrates that he believed so greatly in the medicinal and food values of pure honey that one of the two basic remedies which he used for treatment of nearly all ailments was pure honey; 'hydromel', he called it, mixed with water. Legend says that after his death wild bees swarmed on his tomb and established their home there, and the honey taken therefrom possessed marvellous healing properties. As readers know, I have advised the use of honey as medicine and food throughout this herbal book.

The Greeks, and many peoples since, including the early American settlers, used to plant herbal gardens for use of their families

Conclusion

and animals. Mr. J. E. O'Donovan, of Eire, the greyhound expert and journalist, informed me, in one of his letters to me, that the old-fashioned Irish greyhound breeders very often grew garlic and other herbs for the use of their dogs. I know of several breeders in England, France, and Switzerland, who have already planted former kennel runs with those herbs which they have learned firstly from my books, and then secondly proved with their own dogs, to be of special value in canine diet and medicine.

I would conclude with the quoting of some lines written by my friend, Mr. L. Purcell Weaver, M.A., concerning the naturalistic (cosmotherapy) medicine of Professor Edmond Szekely. For these lines are not inappropriate to describe the naturalistic veterinary medicine detailed in this book, which so many dog breeders are now resolutely following; and which kind of veterinary medicine is closely linked with the natural and true form of human medicine; and which, furthermore, has certainly met with much hostility and opposition. To quote: 'Its revolutionary teachings will be bitterly opposed in high places. It will triumph in the measure that it is true. And it is true in the measure that it heals. This can only be tested by each one giving the system a fair trial for himself and seeing the result. *Qui vivra verra.*'

Appendix

The Herbs in this Book

This appendix is for those who wish to gather their own herbs. Because most of the plants advised in the treatments are so common, no botanical descriptions are given, only the popular and botanical names, enabling readers to look them up in any book on wild flowers, where full descriptions will be given; botanical names are international and are the same in all countries and in all books of wild flowers, only popular names differ. As alternatives are given for many of the herbs in the treatments, those who cannot get one plant will usually be able to find another. A fuller account of these herbs and many others, and where they grow, and their medicinal properties is given in my *Herbal Handbook for Farm and Stable* (Faber and Faber), in the nearly one hundred pages of *materia medica* in that book.

There are three lists: the first are all common weeds, trees, or shrubs growing wild; the second consists of garden plants and herbs; and the third, a few herbs that must mostly be purchased from herbal shops. Nothing is said about the part to be used: that is given in the treatments, Chapter 6. Many health foods stores in England and the United States stock supplies of dried, plain herbs, suitable for canine use.

Once, when the first edition of this canine book appeared, such shops were rare. Now one or more health stores can be found in almost every town in England and America.

COMMON WILD PLANTS

BILBERRY, WHORTLEBERRY. *Vaccinium myrtillus. Vacciniaceae.*

193

The Herbs in this Book

Found on boggy heaths and on mountainsides. Its edible berries are well known.

BLACKBERRY, BRAMBLE. *Rubus fruticosus. Rosaceae.* A common thorny hedgerow and wasteland herb, known for its juicy and edible fruits.

BORAGE. *Borago officinalis. Boraginaceae.* Field and woodland, distinguished by its rough leaves and intensely blue flowers.

BROOM. *Cytisus scoparius. Leguminosae.* Found on dry heaths and sandy soils. Possesses yellow, pea-form flowers.

CHAMOMILE. *Anthemis nobilis. Compositae.* Waste places and damp places. Fragrant, small, daisy-like flowers; very scented, feathery leaves.

CHICKWEED. *Stellaria media. Caryophyllaceae.* A tiny pasture herb with white, starry flowers.

CLOVER (RED). *Trifolium pratense. Leguminosae.* A plant of pastures, with trefoil leaves and globes of red or pink flowers.

COMFREY. *Symphytum officinale. Boraginaceae.* Inhabits ditch-sides, though will also grow in dry places. Now often cultivated as a fodder crop especially in Russia. Large, rough leaves; pinkish or creamy bell-like flowers.

DANDELION. *Taraxacum officinale. Compositae.* Common weed found on waste ground, on banks, and in gardens.

DOCK. *Rumex aquaticus. Polygonum.* A common broad-leaf weed, with spikes of loose, rusty-coloured, reed-like flowers.

ELDER, ELDERBERRY. *Sambucus niger. Caprifoliaceae.* A small tree or shrub, with rich-scented, flat heads of creamy flowers, producing edible black berries.

ELDER, DWARF OR GROUND. *Sambucus ebulus. Caprifoliaceae.* Grows in waste places, is also a persistent garden weed. Resembles a small elder, but its leaves have a stronger odour and its flowers are scentless.

GOOSEGRASS, CLEAVERS. *Galium aparine. Rubiaceae.* A trailing weed with round fruits and square stems, both of clinging nature.

GREATER CELANDINE. *Chelidonium majus. Papaveraceae.* Found by old walls and on rubble, also outskirts of woods. Grey leaves and small, frail, yellow flowers which shed their petals very easily.

HOLLY. *Ilex aquifolium. Aquifoliaceae.* A well-known red-berried bush or tree with prickly leaves.

194

The Herbs in this Book

HOREHOUND. *Marrubium vulgare. Labiatae.* Common in woodland and in hedgerows. Greyish, slightly woolly leaves, spikes of colourless flowers.

IVY. *Hedera helix. Araliaceae.* A well-known evergreen climbing plant with colourless, sweet-scented blossoms. Found on trees, banks, old walls, etc.

MALE FERN. *Aspidium filix-mas. Filices.* Likes woods and shady banks. Distinguished by its tall fern foliage which has numerous scales on the under surface of leaves, and brown spores.

MARSHMALLOW. *Althaea officinalis. Malvaceae.* Of waysides, pink flowers, very round, dark foliage.

MEADOWSWEET. *Spiraea ulmaria. Rosaceae.* Grows in wet meadows. Has rose-form leaves, plumes of creamy, sweet-scented flowers.

NETTLE, STINGING NETTLE. *Urtica diocia. Urticaceae.* A tall perennial, known by its leaves which sting sharply.

OAK. *Quercus robur. Loganiaceae.* A tree of woodlands. Has notable oval fruits in green cups, called acorns.

PLANTAIN. *Plantago major. Plantaginaceae.* Of pastureland and waste places. Distinguished by its flat-growing, oval-shaped and ribbed leaves, and unusual flowering spike, resembling a small bulrush, of greenish-brown hue.

RASPBERRY. *Rubus idaeus. Rosaceae.* A bramble-like woodland shrub, known for its juicy red berries.

THYME. *Thymus vulgaris. Labiatae.* Of moorland and sunny banks. Tiny leaves, the tufts of white-pink flowers of very sweet and aromatic scent.

TOAD-FLAX. *Linaria vulgaris. Scrophulariaceae.* Of pastures and waste places, distinguished by its yellow and cream 'snapdragon' shaped flowers.

VIOLET (SWEET). *Viola odorata. Violaceae.* Of shady banks and woodlands. Well known by its sometimes fragrant, purple flowers. The garden species is also used.

WATERCRESS. *Nasturtium officinale. Cruciferae.* Well-known wild salad plant, growing in running streams, especially spring-water streams. If shop-bought, take care that it does not come from still, copper-sulphated water.

WILD ROSE, SWEET BRIAR. *Rose species. Rosaceae.* A well-known shrub of hedgerow and woodland. Distinguished by its sweet-scented pink flowers and hard, red, shiny, edible fruits—'hips'.

The Herbs in this Book

WOOD-SAGE. *Teucrium scorodonia. Labiatae.* Of shady places and woodlands. Rough, dark leaves, spiky, greenish-yellow, hooded flowers.

YARROW. *Achillea millefolium. Compositae.* A weed of lawns and pastures. Feathery leaves, flat heads of composite, tiny rose or cream-coloured flowers.

GARDEN PLANTS AND HERBS

ASPARAGUS. *Asparagus officinalis. Liliaceae.* Known for its edible shoots. Also found wild.

BALM. *Melissa officinalis. Labiatae.* Hairy leaves, whorls of creamy, hooded flowers: much sought by bees.

CRESS, GARDEN CRESS. *Lepidium sativum. Cruciferae.* The common salad herb with 'hot' leaves.

GARLIC. *Allium sativum. Liliaceae.* Easily grown in gardens or bought from greengrocers. The wild variety grows in damp woodland and pastures.

HOLLYHOCK. *Althea rosea. Malvaceae.* Well known for its tallness and large flowers of various colours with squarish petals.

HYSSOP. *Hyssopus officinalis. Labiatae.* An attractive, very aromatic border plant. Much celebrated in the Bible.

LAVENDER. *Lavandula vera. Labiatae.* Well known, very fragrant when dry or fresh, has small greyish leaves and spikes of blue flowers.

LILY OF THE VALLEY. *Convallaria majalis. Liliaceae.* Well known for its sweet-scented, white flowers; much planted in gardens.

MARIGOLD. *Calendula officinalis. Compositae.* The well-known hardy annual of bright, orange-hued, daisy form or double daisy flowers.

MARJORAM. *Origanum majorana* or *onites. Labiatae.* Very aromatic, of mountain origin, and resembles a tall wild thyme.

MINT. *Mentha viridis. Labiatae.* The common garden salad plant with mint scent.

MUSTARD (BLACK). *Sinapis nigra. Cruciferae.* A common garden weed, with bright yellow flowers and strong-tasting cresslike leaves.

PARSLEY. *Petroselinum hortense. Umbelliferae.* Common garden salad herb, with flat or tightly curled leaves of intense green.

The Herbs in this Book

PEONY. *Paeonia officinalis.* It has distinct solitary red or pink, large, many-petalled flowers, and large, fringed leaves.

POPPY (OPIUM) AND WILD, RED. *Papaver somniferum* and *Papaver rhoeas. Papaveraceae.* The former is a tall plant with grey-blue foliage and big, white-cream flowers; the latter, small, hairy stemmed, with small, brilliant red flowers.

RASPBERRY. (See Wild Herbs.)

ROSEMARY. *Rosmarinus officinalis. Labiatae.* A very aromatic plant of grey-green foliage and small, light blue flowers.

RUE. *Ruta graveolens. Rutaceae.* Distinguished by its much-divided flat, greyish leaves, and small yellow flowers of bitter scent.

SAGE. *Salvia officinalis. Labiatae.* Popular garden culinary herb, also grows in abundance wild, on hills and plains. Grey, strongly scented foliage; spikes of blue flowers.

HERBS TO BE PURCHASED FROM SELLERS

ELM (SLIPPERY), OR RED ELM. *Ulmus fulva. Urticaceae.* The pink-hued very aromatic bark is famous for its medicinal properties.

EUCALYPTUS. *Eucalyptus globulus. Myrtaceae.* This is a sub-tropical tree, distinguished by its tall, graceful form and willow-like foliage. The foliage can be collected in many parts of the Americas, but its extracted oil has to be purchased.

FENUGREEK (SEED). *Trigonella foenum-graecum. Leguminosae.* Sold in some health foods stores.

LIQUORICE. *Glycyrrhiza glabra. Leguminosae.* The root can be bought from herbalists or the black solid juice (usually called Spanish Liquorice) is sold in sticks.

SKULLCAP. *Scutellaria lateriflora. Labiatae.* The dried herb is procurable from most herbalists.

SENNA. *Cassia acutifolia. Leguminosae.* Its foliage and flat seed-pods are sold by most herbalists and some chemists.

WITCH HAZEL. *Hamamelis virginiana. Hamamelidaceae.* The bark is sold by herbalists, also its extract in alcohol. Most chemists sell the astringent extract.

PROPRIETARY HERBAL PRODUCTS. Freshly dried and compressed herbs in tablet form, as mentioned in this book, garlic and rue tablets ('Herbal compound'), wild raspberry, seaweed and

The Herbs in this Book

comfrey minerals, and other blended powdered herbs and tree barks, also herbal insecticide herbs, made to my own formulae, can all be obtained by post. As there is still no fixed address in either England or the U.S.A. the present address, and lists of products available, can be obtained from Mrs. J. N. Levy, 642 Wilmslow Road, Didsbury, Manchester 20, England.

Index

Abrasions, 102
Abscesses, 102–3
Afterbirth, retained, 58
Afghans, 7, 26, 32, 39, 53–4, 77, 84,
    85, 104, 108, 132, 137, 139, 148,
    152, 154, 155, 168, 186, 188, 190
Ailments, *see* Diseases
Ajman kennels, 155
Alsatians, 51, 166
Anaemia, 103
Anal glands trouble, 103
Ancylostomiasis, *see* Hook worms
Appetite, depraved, 24, 82
Appetite, loss of, 103–4
'Arabian' cakes, 33
Arabian greyhounds, *see* Salukis
Arabian horses, 50
Arctic sleigh dogs, 21, 31
Areca nuts, 176–7
Arriman (cat), 97
Arthritis, 104
Artichoke, 36, 113
Average-size dog, defined, 92
Avocado oil, 42

Bad breath, 104
Baldness, 105
Baldwin, James, 182
Balk-Roesch, Mrs. Helen, 143
Ballykelly Irish Wolfhounds and
    Deerhounds, 108
Bancroft-Wilson, Mrs. S., 57
Barber, Mrs. Winifred, 68

Barley, 35, 66
Beagles, 122
Beans, in diet, 36
Béchamp, Antoine, 126
Bee herbs, 40
Beta haemolytic streptococcus
    (b. h. s.), *see* Streptococcal infec-
    tions
Bitches, *see* In-whelp bitches, care of
Bladder troubles, 105–6
Bleeding of wounds, 106–8
Boc, Baron de, 122
Bones in diet, 22, 28, 30, 44, 48
Border Collies, 34, 51–2
Boredom, 62; *see* Hysteria
Borzois, 23, 53, 111, 148
Boxers, 124
Breast tumours, 108–9
Brock, D. W. E., 26
Broken bones, *see* Limbs, fractures of
Bronchitis, 109, 148, *see also* Pneu-
    monia
Brood bitches, care of, 48, 62–4; *see
    also* In-whelp bitches
Broomleaf Cockers, England, 160
Brown, Peggy E., 51–2
Bull terriers, 51
Buried meat, 26–7
Burns, *see* Scalds
Butter, in diet, 38
Buttermilk, in diet, 37–8
Butterworth, Mrs. Betty (Madame
    Coigny), 120–2

Index

Index

Index

Index

Index

Index

Index

Index